YOU ARE WHAT YOU EAT.

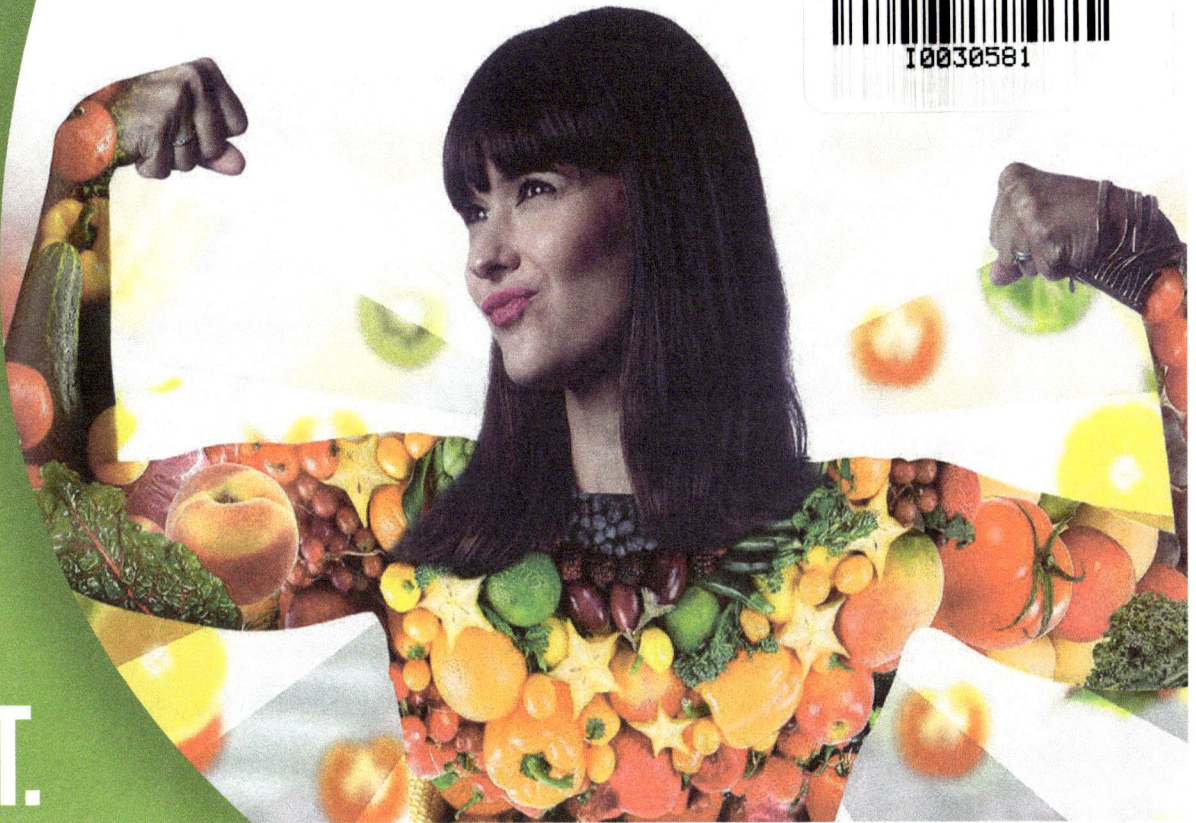

Every 28 days, your skin replaces itself. Your liver, 5 months. Your bones, 10 years. Your body makes new cells through the nutrition you give it. What you consume literally becomes you. Given proper nutrition, the human body has the amazing ability to heal itself. To do so, a healthy diet is required. We can't realistically expect that if we eat junk, our bodies will sustain proper health and healing.

Most lifestyle changes, especially ones dealing with health and nutrition, can be quite overwhelming. Human beings are creatures of habit. It can be challenging to change our ingrained habits. At the West Clinic, we know this and want to assist you in this transition. In this section of your book, you will find diet and exercise programs that, if purchased, will provide you with the guidance, information, and assistance you will need in order to change your habits and your overall health.

Those who think they have no time for healthy eating and exercise, will sooner or later have to make time for illness.

The following pages contain meal planning tips and recipes to assist you in your journey toward achieving and maintaining optimal health.

TIPS TO HEALTHY EATING

KEYS TO SUCCESS

Timing is Important!
- Eat within 30-60 minutes of waking.
- Always eat 1-2 hours before working out.
- Eat every 2-3 hours and no longer than 3 hours.
- Eat 5-7 times a day (i.e., 7a.m., 10a.m., 1p.m., 4p.m., 7p.m., 10p.m.).
- NO STARVING! Fire up that metabolism!

Watch Your Serving Size!
- Each meal should be no less than 200 calories; aim for 300 calories each.
- It is important to watch your serving size with most foods, especially fats, carbohydrates, and high calorie proteins. For example, it's easy to eat more than one serving of lean proteins such as chicken breast and cottage cheese.
- You can eat as many vegetables as you would like, but at least 4-5 servings per day.
- Eat 1-3 servings of fruit each day.

Meal Balance is Key!
- Three of the five meals should have protein, carbohydrates, and a mono- and/or polyunsaturated fat.
- The last meal could be just a protein (i.e., cottage cheese or chicken breast).
- Try not eat whole grains for the last one or two meals. For example, after 4:30p.m., eat vegetables and/or fruit instead of bread, pasta, or rice.
- Try not to eat carbohydrates alone (i.e., apple with almond butter).

Prepare Ahead of Time!
- Make sure you have healthy choices on hand.
- Pack healthy, balanced meals for work.
- Bring healthy foods when you are out-and-about (i.e., protein bars, nuts, and fruit).
- Cook in bulk and make use of portable storage containers.
- PREPARE, OR PREPARE TO FAIL!

Tips To Consider!
- Eat organic when you can, especially the "dirty dozen".
- Some people benefit from allergy free food living (i.e., gluten, dairy). For specific food sensitivities, consider getting tested.
- Learn you caloric needs.
- Exercise 30 minutes daily.
- Get 7-9 hours a sleep at night.
- Take important supplements (i.e., Omega-3 Fish Oil, Vitamin D, Probiotic).

TO AVOID:
- Refined carbohydrates (i.e. enriched and bleached white flour)
- Added sugars
- Sugar substitutes (i.e..Splenda, Aspartame, Saccharin, etc.)
- High sodium foods
- Hydrogenated oils and trans-fats
- High fructose corn syrup and maltodextrin
- Foods high in saturated fats
- Processed foods
- MSG

HYDRATION:
- Drink water, skim milk, green tea, and plain black coffee.
- Drink of minimum of 64 ounces of water each day; you may need more depending on your body weight.
- Bring a water bottle with you wherever you go.
- Drink a glass of water before each meal and one while eatin

MEAL PLANNING

PROTEIN:

Salmon (3-6 oz., 2/week)
Lean Steaks (4-6 oz., 2/week)
Pork Tenderloin (4-6 oz., 2/week)
Tuna
Seafood (shrimp, crab, scallops, fish)
Lean Ground Turkey or Chicken

Fat Free Cottage Cheese
Fat Free Greek Yogurt
Skim, Almond, Rice, Soy Milk Chicken Breast 100% Whey Protein
Beans and Legumes
Tofu
Eggs Chicken Sausage

Protein should be 30-40% of Daily Calorie Intake.

CARBS:

Brown Rice
Whole Wheat Pasta
100% Whole Wheat Bread
Organic Bread (Men's or Hemp Bread)
Couscous
Quinoa
Oatmeal/Old Fashioned Oats

La Tortilla (7g pro, 50 kcal)
Fresh/Frozen Fruit
Fresh/Frozen Vegetables
Sweet Potatoes or Yams
Natural Granola
Kashi (crackers, cereal, bars)
Triscuits

Have 1-2servings of whole grain carbohydrates a day. The other 4-5 servings should be from fruits and vegetables. Carbohydrates should be 30-40% of Daily Calorie Intake.

HEART HEALTHY FATS:

Raw, unsalted nuts: almonds, walnuts, soy nuts
Avocadoes
Hummus
Olive, Grape Seed, and Walnut Oils

Natural Peanut Butter
Fat Free/Reduced Fat Cheese
Flax Seed or Flax Seed Oil

Have 3 servings of Heart Healthy Fats a day. Healthy Fats should be 20-30% of Daily Calorie Intake.

WEST CLINIC PLAN

PHASE 1 will get your metabolism reset and activated to start the deep mobilization of fat stores and increase your lean muscle. It will retrain your taste palate to not crave the sweet calorie rich and nutrition void foods. It also aims at detoxifying the body and getting the liver more effective and efficient at eliminating toxins. **PHASE 1** lasts for two weeks, but can be followed for up to four weeks. This phase provides for the most rapid weight loss.

PHASE 2 can be started upon completion of reaching your **PHASE 1** goal. It allows for more types of foods and a friendlier family structure. Foods such as dairy and grains will be carefully reintroduced into the diet one at a time to watch for sensitivity reactions. The weight loss rates will not be as rapid as **PHASE 1**, but that is a normal part of adding new foods to your diet. **PHASE 2** is exciting as foods will be bursting with robust flavor as they can be prepared with great spices and flavor.

Once you reach your weight goal, you will enter the maintenance phase or **PHASE 3**. This phase allows for all foods to fit but with more awareness and understanding of your food choices and their effects on your weight and health. If you find yourself gaining weight, not feeling well, or frequently fatigued, you can always go back to **PHASE 1** or **PHASE 2** to get back to the goal you once reached through a healthy meal plan garnished with exercise.

Those in PHASE 1 should stick to only **PHASE 1 recipes,

PHASE 2 can use **PHASE 1** and **PHASE 2** recipes,

And **PHASE 3** can use any of the recipes in this book (phases 1-3).**

CONTENTS

PHASE 1

THE WEST CLINIC 4 LIFE PLAN IS A VERY HEALTHY, CLEAN WAY OF EATING AND LIVING. YOU ARE ALLOWED TO STAY ON THIS TYPE OF CLEAN EATING AS LONG AS YOU WANT. THE HEALTH BENEFITS ARE IMMENSE AND WELL-STUDIED WITH THIS PLAN. PHASE 1 IS A GREAT TOOL FOR GETTING STARTED. IF YOU FEEL YOU ARE NOT GETTING ENOUGH CALORIES OR FEELING TIRED, THEN PHASE 2 IS THE NEXT STEP AFTER 2-4 WEEKS OF PHASE 1. PHASE 1 IS NOT MEANT TO STARVE YOU; IT IS DESIGNED TO DETOXIFY THE BODY AND TO BREAK THE UNHEALTHY EATING HABITS AND FOOD ADDICTIONS. YOUR METABOLIC TEST AND NUTRITION CONSULT WITH THE DIETITIAN WILL HELP GIVE YOU AN OVERVIEW OF WHAT NUTRIENTS ARE NEEDED FOR YOU TO FUNCTION AT YOUR BEST.

PHASE 1 TIPS AND OVERVIEW

1. Eat low glycemic index (GI) foods to keep blood sugars steady and insulin low to help prevent fat storage.

2. H20: You need to drink ½ body weight in ounces throughout the day. H20 is vital to weight loss, cell hydration, and optimal function. Use filtered water (i.e. Brita filter) to take out unneeded fluoride and other chemicals.

3. Vegetables and fruits: refer the list of acceptable foods. The lower the glycemic index of the food the better for decreasing insulin spikes and blood sugar levels. More nutrition will be consumed from the food if it is not over cooked. Eat in a steamed or raw state and avoid over cooking (boiled, baked or over fried).

4. Lean and clean meats (organic if possible): refer the list of acceptable foods. Healthy meats are your source of amino acids to stimulate muscle repair and development, as well as increase fat loss. Consuming smaller animal proteins like chicken and fish more often than larger animals like beef will be helpful. The reason for that is large animals have a large amount of hormones in their meat and fat that can lead to weight gain. Even if organic, they are thousand pound animals and will have a large amounts of unwanted estrogens and other hormones that can lead to weight gain.

5. Eggs: egg whites only during PHASE 1. You can also use Egg White Egg Beaters®.

1. Avoid stimulants like caffeinated tea, coffee, chocolate or cigarettes as these will increase carbohydrate absorption rates of foods and increase insulin resistance.

2. Do not eat processed or packaged foods. Instead choose low sugar protein bars as an on the go food.

3. Do not eat fast foods. Quality food ordered out is acceptable if they meet the meal plan guidelines.

4. Do not eat or drink dairy. Dairy can be an inflammatory food. It has high animal hormone content.
The lactose sugar will cause an insulin spike that leads to weight gain. It also decreases your thyroid hormone and slows metabolism.

5. No sugar, artificial sweeteners, or products containing them. Stevia in moderation is ok, but do not over sweeten food as the goal is to decrease sweet cravings and retrain the taste palate to less sweet foods. Studies show drinking artificially sweetened drinks leads to weight gain NOT weight loss. It is also important to stay away from fruit juices or soda. Eat whole fruits instead to get all the fiber, antioxidants and nutrients the way nature intended.

6. Do not consume alcohol. It slows down the metabolism and has nutrition void calories.

7. Go organic when you can:
   - Meats (added hormones and high Omega 6 fats make weight loss difficult)
   - Fruits and veggies that you eat with a skin (i.e. apples, grapes, berries)

Herbicides and pesticides on skin can't be washed off and affect health/weight.

MEAL PLAN

BREAKFAST:

Fiber- 15 grams prior to meal
Water
1 Protein
1 Fruits
1 Veggie
1 Healthy fat or nut

10 AM SNACK*

Water
Protein shake (mixed in cold water) 1 Fruit

LUNCH:

Water
1 Protein
2Veggies
1 Healthy fat or nut

3PM SNACK*

Water
1 Healthy fat or nut 1 Protein

DINNER

Water
Fiber- 15 grams prior to meal 1 Protein
2-4 Veggies
1 Healthy fat or nut

BEDTIME SNACK- *within an hour of going to sleep*

Protein shake or 1 Protein
½ Healthy fat or nut

If working out, you can do your serving of fruit prior to the workout for extra energy.
Can substitute approved protein/meal replacement bar for on the go nutrition (discuss with trainer).

HERE IS MEAL PLAN SAMPLE AND RECIPES TO PROVIDE YOU GUIDANCE IN MAKING FOOD CHOICES DURING PHASE 1. YOU DO NOT HAVE TO FOLLOW THIS EXACT MEAL PLAN AND YOU CAN SUBSTITUTE OTHER MEALS FROM PHASE 1. USE THIS MEAL PLAN AS A TOOL TO HELP YOU MAKE CLEAN EATING CHOICES.

WEST CLINIC 4 LIFE PHASE 1:
1 MONTH OF EASY EATING WEEK 1

Sunday	Monday	Tuesday	Wednesday	Thursday	Friday	Saturday
Meal 1 So Spicy Omelet (pg 15)	Meal 1 Smoothie (pg 19-20)	Meal 1 Egg whites with spinach	Meal 1 Protein Shake Fruit	Meal 1 Simple Omelet (pg 15)	Meal 1 Avocado and Fruit Salad (pg 32)	Meal 1 Zucchini Scrambled Eggs (pg 16)
Meal 2 Avocado Fruit Salad (pg 32)	Meal 2 Leftover Kale Chips	Meal 2 Fruit Walnuts	Meal 2 Almonds 1 Hard Boiled Egg	Meal 2 Smoothie (pg 19-20)	Meal 2 Lettuce Wrap (pg 46-47)	Meal 2 Sweet and Spicy Apples and Sweet Potatoes (pg 60)
Meal 3 Vegetable	Meal 3 Leftover chicken	Meal 3 Tomato Salad (pg 56)	Meal 3 Tasty Tuna Salad (pg 40)	Meal 3 Tomato Cucumber Salad (pg 57)	Meal 3 Not Your Average Chicken Salad (pg 33)	Meal 3 Spinach Salad (pg 27)
Meal 4 Chicken (pg 33-38) Sweet potatoes (pg 61)	Meal 4 Salad (pg 27-33)	Meal 4 Almond Flax Pizza (pg 48)	Meal 4 Salad (pg 27-33)	Meal 4 Warm S pinach Chicken Salad (pg 27)	Meal 4 Protein Shake	Meal 4 Guacamole Turkey Patties (pg 40)
Meal 5 Crispy Kale Chips (pg 60)	Meal 5 Protein Shake	Meal 5 Vegetable	Meal 5 Leftover Pizza	Meal 5 Walnuts	Meal 5 Almond Broccoli Salad (pg 58)	Meal 5 Fruit
			Meal 6 Vegetable			

WEST CLINIC 4 LIFE PHASE 1:
1 MONTH OF EASY EATING WEEK 2

Sunday	Monday	Tuesday	Wednesday	Thursday	Friday	Saturday
Meal 1 Avocado Egg Salad (pg 31)	Meal 1 Smoothie (pg 19-20)	Meal 1 Protein Shake Fruit	Meal 1 Simple Omelet (pg 15)	Meal 1 Spanish Scrambled Eggs (pg 17)	Meal 1 Smoothie (pg 19-20)	Meal 1 Veggie Breakfast Hash Browns (pg 18)
Meal 2 Fruit	Meal 2 Vegetable Almonds	Meal 2 Vegetable 1 Hard Boiled Egg	Meal 2 Smoothie (pg 19-20)	Meal 2 Fruit	Meal 2 Vegetable	Meal 2 Fruit Walnuts
Meal 3 Mini Kale Burgers (pg 39)	Meal 3 Leftover Avocado Egg Salad	Meal 3 Leftover Mini Kale Burgers	Meal 3 Salad (pg 27-33)	Meal 3 Leftover Tomato Chicken	Meal 3 Lettuce Taco (pg 46) Pico de Gallo (pg 49)	Meal 3 Soup (pg 21-26)
Meal 4 Salad (pg 27-33)	Meal 4 Crispy Kale Chips (pg 60)	Meal 4 Salad (pg 27-33)	Meal 4 Skillet Tomato Chicken (pg 37)	Meal 4 Salad (pg 27-33)	Meal 4 Protein Shake	Meal 4 Rosemary Chicken and Potatoes (pg 38)
Meal 5 Crispy Kale Chips (pg 60)	Meal 5 Chicken (pg 33-38)	Meal 5 Eggplant Tuna Salad (pg 41)	Meal 5 Leftover Tuna Salad	Meal 5 Lemon Roasted Peppers (pg 59)	Meal 5 Grilled Chicken Breast	Meal 5 Tomato Salad (pg 56)
			Meal 6 Leftover Kale Chips	Meal 6 Protein Shake (if hungry)	Meal 6 Roasted Florets and Peppers (pg 59)	

WEST CLINIC 4 LIFE PHASE 1:
1 MONTH OF EASY EATING WEEK 3

Sunday	Monday	Tuesday	Wednesday	Thursday	Friday	Saturday
Meal 1 Veggie Egg Scramble (pg 16)	Meal 1 So Spicy Omelet (pg 15)	Meal 1 Smoothie (pg 19-20)	Meal 1 Veggie Breakfast Hash Browns (pg 18)	Meal 1 Egg whites with spinach and peppers	Meal 1 Protein Shake Fruit	Meal 1 Spicy Breakfast Patties (pg 18)
Meal 2 Fruit	Meal 2 Smoothie (pg 19-20)	Meal 2 2 Hard Boiled Eggs	Meal 2 Tomato Avocado Tartar (pg 57)	Meal 2 Sweet and Spicy Apples and Sweet Potatoes (pg 60)	Meal 2 Leftover Pizza	Meal 2 Avocado Fruit Salad (pg 32)
Meal 3 Leftover Rosemary Chicken and Potatoes	Meal 3 Leftover Salmon	Meal 3 Leftover Pomegranate Pork	Meal 3 Smoothie (pg 19-20)	Meal 3 Shrimp (pg 43-45)	Meal 3 Crispy Kale Chips (pg 60)	Meal 3 2 Hard Boiled Eggs
Meal 4 Salad (pg 27-33)	Meal 4 Salad (pg 27-33)	Meal 4 Vegetable Walnuts	Meal 4 Chicken (pg 33-38)	Meal 4 Almond Flax Pizza (pg 48)	Meal 4 Chicken Salad (pg 33)	Meal 4 Warm Veggie Salad (pg 58)
Meal 5 Salmon (pg 41-42)	Meal 5 Pomegranate Pork (pg 39)	Meal 5 Lettuce Taco (pg 46) Pico de Gallo (pg 49)	Meal 5 Spinach Salad (pg 27)	Meal 5 Vegetable	Meal 5 Almond Broccoli Salad (pg 58)	Meal 5 Leftover Kale Chips
Meal 6 Protein Shake	Meal 6 Vegetable Almonds					

WEST CLINIC 4 LIFE PHASE 1:
1 MONTH OF EASY EATING WEEK 4

Sunday	Monday	Tuesday	Wednesday	Thursday	Friday	Saturday
Meal 1 Simple Omelet (pg 15)	Meal 1 Zucchini Scrambled Eggs (pg 16)	Meal 1 Protein Shake Fruit	Meal 1 Spanish Egg Scramble (pg 17)	Meal 1 Zucchini Frittata (pg 17)	Meal 1 Smoothie (pg 19-20)	Meal 1 Veggie Breakfast Hash Browns (pg 18)
Meal 2 Protein Shake	Meal 2 Vegetable Almonds	Meal 2 Avocado Egg Salad (pg 31)	Meal 2 Avocado Fruit Salad (pg 32)	Meal 2 Tomato Cucumber Salad (pg 57)	Meal 2 2 Hard Boiled Eggs	Meal 2 Smoothie (pg 19-20)
Meal 3 Guacamole Turkey Patties (pg 40)	Meal 3 Smoothie (pg 19-20)	Meal 3 Chicken (pg 33-38) Roasted Florets and Peppers (pg 59)	Meal 3 Leftover Chicken	Meal 3 Salmon (pg 41-42)	Meal 3 Almond Broccoli Salad (pg 58)	Meal 3 Mini Kale Turkey Burgers (pg 39)
Meal 4 Salad (pg 27-33)	Meal 4 Lettuce Taco (pg 46) with Leftover Guacamole	Meal 4 Salad (pg 27-33)	Meal 4 Warm Veggie Salad (pg 58)	Meal 4 Salad (pg 27-33)	Meal 4 Chicken (pg 33-38) Sweet Potato Fries (pg 61)	Meal 4 Salad (pg 27-33)
Meal 5 Fruit Walnuts	Meal 5 Spinach Red/ Green Peppers Oil and vinegar	Meal 5 Egg whites Sweet Peppers	Meal 5 Shrimp Lettuce Wrap (pg 47)	Meal 5 Protein Shake	Meal 5 Fruit	Meal 5 Avocado and tomatoes
			Meal 6 Protein Shake	Meal 6 Walnuts		

Simple Omelet

4-5 egg whites

1 egg yolk

2 Tbsp. almond or rice milk

1 plum or Roma tomato, chopped

2 Tbsp. garlic, minced

1 cup firmly packed spinach, shredded

2 Tbsp. red onion, minced

3 slices of turkey or lean meat

1/3 cup bell pepper (any color), chopped

Olive oil-based cooking spray

Beat egg whites with the yolk and almond/rice milk.

Quick sauté the vegetables until soft.

Pour eggs into a small frying pan coated with cooking spray. Cook until firm. Add vegetables on one half of omelet, and then fold other half over top. Let sit for 30 seconds or so, then serve.

So Spicy Omelet

INGREDIENTS

4 egg whites (organic)

2oz can green chilies, drained and chopped

1 tsp olive oil

Cayenne pepper to taste

Ground pepper to taste

Beat egg whites and chilies in a medium bowl.

In a small frying pan over low-medium heat, add olive oil, eggs/chilies, and Cayenne pepper and ground pepper to taste. When eggs are firm and cooked through, fold half over top.

Zucchini Scrambled Eggs

INGREDIENTS

2 Egg whites (organic)

1 whole egg (organic)

1 cup red bell pepper, diced

½ cup onion, diced

1 ½ cups zucchini, diced

2 tsp olive oil

Ground black pepper to taste

Sauté vegetables in medium pan until almost tender.

In a bowl, whisk egg and egg whites. Pour eggs over vegetables and continue cooking and stirring until eggs are cooked through. Add pepper to taste.

Veggie Egg Scramble

INGREDIENTS

1 ½ cups asparagus, chopped

¼ cup chopped onion

2 cloves garlic, minced

1 cup chopped mushrooms

3 cups spinach

6 egg whites

2 Roma tomatoes, diced

2 tsp olive oil

Ground pepper to taste

Blanche asparagus - in a medium pan, bring water to a boil, add asparagus and boil for about 2 minutes. Remove immediately and place in a bowl of cold water until cooled.

In a large skillet over medium heat, sauté in olive oil the onion, garlic, and mushrooms until tender. Add spinach and asparagus. Cook until spinach is wilted (3-5 minutes). Add and stir in egg whites and tomatoes. Scramble and cook for about 3-5 minutes. Add ground pepper to taste.

Spanish Scrambled Eggs

INGREDIENTS

4 egg whites

½ tsp dried oregano

½ tsp paprika

½ tsp ground pepper

1 zucchini, julienned

1 Roma tomato, diced

1 red bell pepper, diced

½ onion, chopped

2 tsp olive oil

In a medium bowl, whisk egg whites, oregano, paprika and ground pepper.

In a large skillet, sauté in olive oil the zucchini, bell pepper, tomato, and onion on high heat for about 3 minutes or until vegetables are soft. Drizzle eggs over top and continue cooking until egg whites are cooked.

Eating healthy is a sign of self-love and self-respect.

Zucchini Frittata

INGREDIENTS

6 egg whites (organic)

¼ cup chopped parsley

2 cups diced zucchini

1 onion, chopped

1 clove garlic, minced

2 Tbsp. olive oil

In a large bowl, combine all ingredients except oil and mix well.

Heat oil in large skillet over medium heat. Add egg mixture and cook until golden brown on bottom, then flip and cook other side until golden. Cut into wedges before serving.

Veggie Breakfast Hash Browns

INGREDIENTS

5 red potatoes, unpeeled and diced

1 squash, peeled and diced

1 tsp Rosemary

½ tsp ground pepper

3 Tbsp. olive oil

2 shallots, chopped

1 head of broccoli, chopped

1 cup chopped sweet peppers (your choice of color)

1/3 cup chopped red bell pepper

Heat oven to 425°

On a baking sheet, place potatoes and squash. Drizzle olive oil, rosemary, and black pepper over the top. Bake for 25 minutes or until potatoes are tender.

In a large skillet over medium-high heat, sauté shallots, broccoli, bell pepper and sweet pepper for about 1-2 minutes. Add potato-squash mixtures and cook for about 5 minutes all together.

Spicy Breakfast Patties

INGREDIENTS

1 lb ground turkey

½ cup minced onion

¼ cup chopped basil

¼ cup chopped parsley

2 cloves garlic, minced

½ tsp dried thyme

1 tsp red pepper flakes

1 tsp ground pepper

2 egg whites (organic)

2 Tbsp.. olive oil

In a large mixing bowl, combine and mix all ingredients except for olive oil. Shape into flat patties.

In a large skillet over medium heat, heat oil and cook patties on both sides until cooked through.

Tropical Smoothie

Puree all ingredients.

INGREDIENTS

1 handful spinach leaves

½ banana

½ peeled orange

1 cup pineapple, diced

½ cup blueberries

1 scoop whey protein powder

1-2 cups water

Handful of ice cubes

Vitamin Pro Smoothie

Puree all ingredients.

INGREDIENTS

½ cup alfalfa sprouts

¼ cup frozen strawberries

¼ cup frozen mixed berries

¼ cup frozen mango

1 ½ tsp. flax oil

1 scoop whey protein powder

1 cup cold water

Handful of ice cubes

Kale Berry Blend Smoothie

INGREDIENTS

1 heaping cup of Kale

½ cup raspberries

½ cup blackberries

1/2 cup pineapple, diced

3-4 strawberries

1 scoop whey protein powder

1 cup cold water

Handful of ice cubes

Puree all ingredients.

Berry Boost Blast

INGREDIENTS

½ cup blueberries

½ cup raspberries

5 almonds, chopped

1 Tbsp. ground flaxseed

1 scoop vanilla whey protein

1 cup cold water

Handful of ice cubes

Puree all ingredients.

Avocado Lime Smoothie

INGREDIENTS

½ avocado, peeled and pitted

2 limes, 1 squeezed and 1 peeled

1 scoop vanilla protein powder

½ cup almond milk

½ Tbsp. vanilla extract

Handful of ice cubes

Puree all ingredients.

Cold Vegetable Soup

INGREDIENTS

½ cup red wine vinegar

½ cup olive oil

5 large ripe tomatoes, chopped

1 ½ cups canned tomato juice

2 eggs (organic), lightly beaten

2 red bell peppers, seeded and chopped

2 onions, chopped

1 shallot, chopped

2 cucumbers, peeled and sliced

1 tsp cayenne pepper

1 tsp ground pepper

¼ cup chopped dill

In a small bowl, whisk vinegar, olive oil, tomato juice, and eggs.

Puree vegetables in small batches in blender or food processor. Add tomato juice mixture to help puree more smoothly. Vegetables do not have to be pureed completely.

Pour pureed vegetables into a large bowl and add cayenne, ground pepper, and dill. Mix ingredients. Chill for at least 4 hours before serving.

Spicy Ginger Soup

INGREDIENTS

4 cups reduced-sodium (organic) chicken broth

1 ½ cups cilantro

2-inch knob of fresh ginger, unpeeled

2 ½ cloves garlic

1 Thai chili pepper

1 lb. fresh-cooked shrimp peeled and deveined, or chicken

1 cup Asian-style vegetables, can use frozen bag

Pour chicken broth into a microwave-safe bowl and microwave covered on high until broth is hot, approximately 3 minutes, depending on the power of your appliance.

Meanwhile, chop cilantro, including stems. Reserve 1 cup of chopped leaves for garnish. Thinly slice ginger. Crush garlic cloves with the flat side of your knife. Cut chili pepper in half; remove seeds if you want less heat in your soup.

When broth is hot, pour into a medium saucepan. Add chopped cilantro stems and leaves (except reserved cup), ginger, garlic and chili pepper and cover. Simmer over medium heat for 5 minutes.

Strain broth into the microwave-safe bowl, and then return strained broth to saucepan. Add shrimp and vegetables. Cook for 3 minutes. Garnish with cilantro leaves you've set aside and discard the rest.

SERVES
4

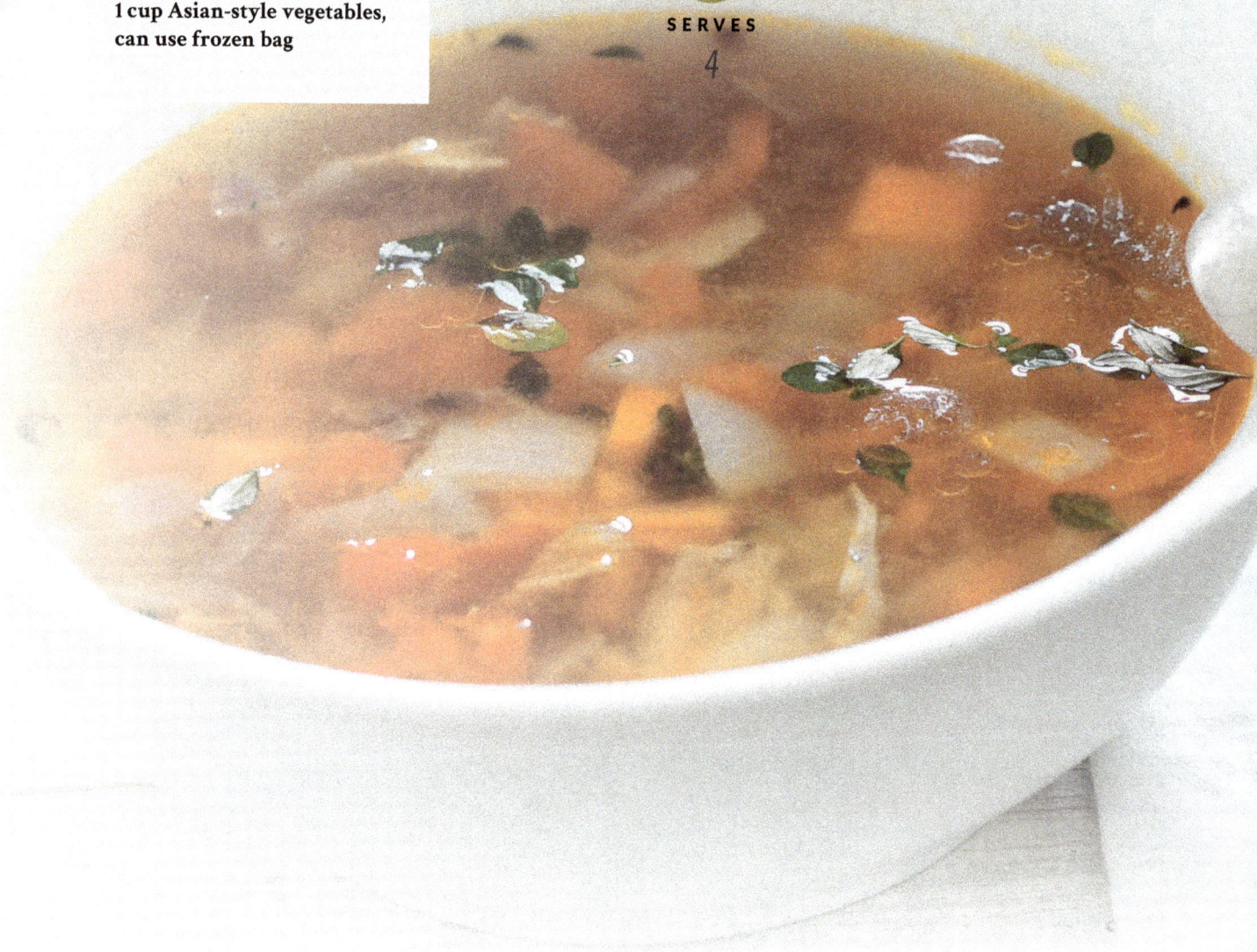

Tofu and Chicken Soup

INGREDIENTS

1 Tbsp. garlic, minced

2 tsp. olive oil

3 ½ cups low-sodium (organic) chicken broth

3 Tbsp. rice vinegar

2 Tbsp. Braggs Amino Acid

½ tsp. crushed red pepper flakes

14 ounce package of extra firm tofu cut into small cubes

1 ½ cups of cooked shredded chicken breast

1 cup shredded cabbage or coleslaw mix

¼ cup eggbeaters or egg whites

1 tsp. sesame oil

In a large pot sauté garlic in hot oil over medium heat. Add in broth, vinegar, Braggs, and red pepper flakes. Bring to a boil.

Add in chicken and tofu, lower heat and simmer. Add eggbeaters/egg whites, stirring to mix. Add cabbage and remove from heat.

Stir in sesame oil. Add extra rice vinegar to personal taste. Sliced mushrooms may be added when sautéing garlic.

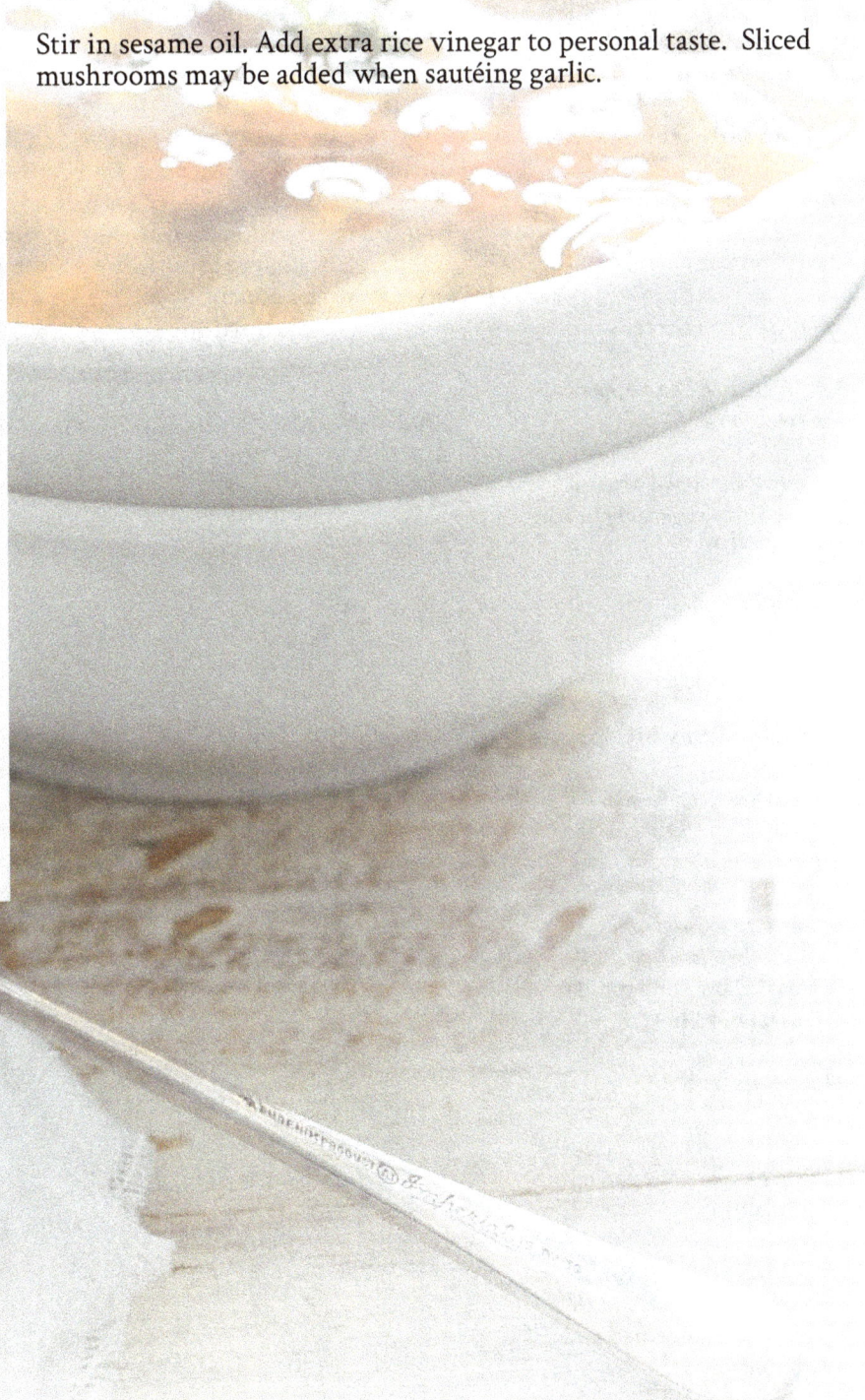

Seafood Soup

INGREDIENTS

¼ cup extra-virgin olive oil

1 medium-size Spanish onion, cut into ½-inch dice

8 cloves garlic, thinly sliced

3 Tbsp. tomato paste

2 tsp. fresh thyme leaves

¼ tsp. saffron threads

1 tsp. crushed red pepper flakes

1 ¼ cups "certified organic" low-sodium vegetable broth diluted with

1 ¼ cups water

1 ½ cups dry white wine

¼ cup distilled white vinegar

3 medium-size plum tomatoes, coarsely chopped, with their juice

1 cup tomato juice

18 small clams, or 9 regular clams (about 1 lb.) *

12 mussels (about 12 oz.) , bearded *

1 ½ lb. bass or snapper, cut in 1-inch cubes

6 medium-size to large shrimp (about 6 oz.), with tails, peeled, deveined and cut in half lengthwise

1 Tbsp. extra-virgin olive oil

3 Tbsp. fresh flat-leaf parsley leaves, chopped

Heat the olive oil in a heavy-bottomed soup pot over medium heat. Add the onion and garlic and cook until softened but not browned, about 4 minutes.

Add the tomato paste, thyme, saffron, and red pepper flakes. Cook and stir to coat the other ingredients with the tomato paste for about 3 minutes.

Add the vegetable broth diluted with 1 ¼ cups water, wine, vinegar, tomatoes, tomato juice, and bring to a simmer, then lower the heat and let simmer for 15 minutes.

Add the clams and mussels, submerging them with a spoon, and cook, uncovered, until they open, about 5 minutes; discard any that do not open. Add the fish and shrimp to the pot, gently poaching them until the fish is opaque and the shrimp are firm and pink, 3 to 4 minutes.

Divide the stew among 6 wide, shallow bowls. Drizzle some olive oil and scatter some parsley over each serving.

* Scrubbed under cold running water.

SERVES

6

You only get one body in this life. There are no trade-ins or upgrades. Don't abuse your body by feeding it garbage. Enrich it with nutrients your body needs to THRIVE, not just SURVIVE.

Colorful Chicken Thai Soup

INGREDIENTS

2 Tbsp. extra-virgin olive oil

1 clove garlic, minced

1 medium onion, chopped

1 cup carrots, chopped into ½ -inch pieces

1 cup small white or red potatoes, chopped into ½ -inch pieces

Sea salt and ground black pepper, to taste

1 ½ cups low-sodium (organic) chicken broth

½ cup light coconut milk

½ cup almond or rice milk

2 boneless, skinless chicken breasts (4 ounces each)

½ cup snow peas, cut lengthwise

2 tsp. red chili pepper flakes (or to taste)

1 Tbsp. curry paste (such as Thai Kitchen)

2 tsp. fresh lemon juice

4 Tbsp. cilantro, coarsely chopped

Heat oil in a pot over medium heat. Add garlic, onion, carrots, and potatoes. Season with salt and pepper and sauté until onions are lightly translucent.

Add broth and coconut and milks. Bring to a light boil.

Add chicken, cover and let simmer for 12 minutes over medium-low to medium heat.

Remove chicken and set aside. Add snow peas, chili flakes, and curry paste to soup. Simmer for 2-3 minutes.

When cool enough to handle, slice chicken and add pieces back to the soup.

Season with additional salt and pepper, if desired. Add lemon juice, sprinkle in cilantro, and serve.

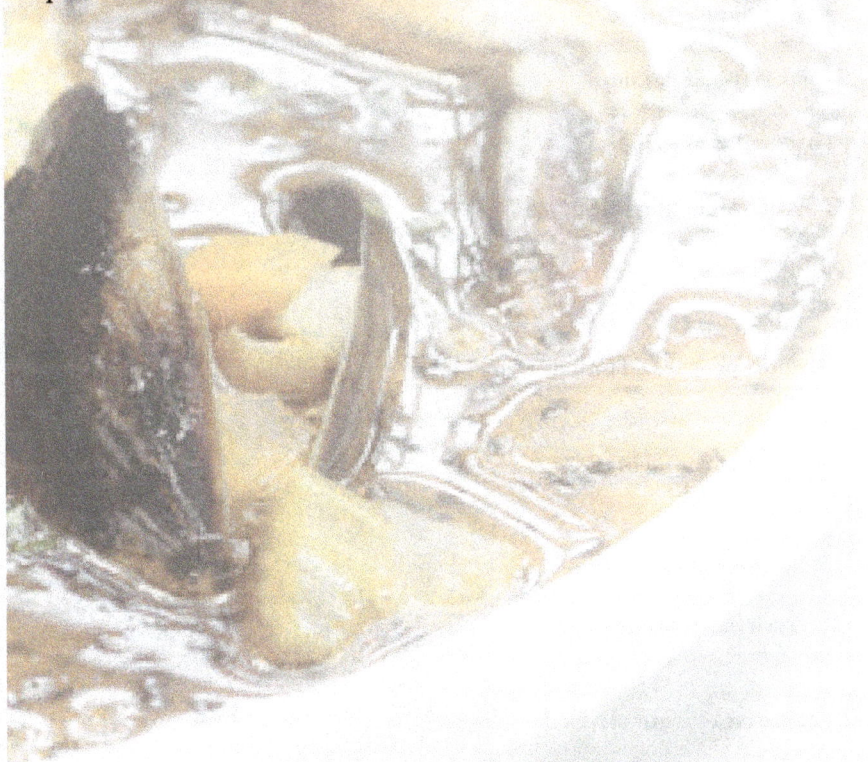

Avocado Scallop Soup

INGREDIENTS

2 cups plum tomatoes, chopped

1 cup cucumber, peeled, seeded, and chopped

¾ cup roasted red pepper, chopped

1/3 cup celery, chopped

½ cup scallions, chopped

3 Tbsp. whole cilantro

1 Tbsp. flat-leaf parsley

1 Tbsp. red wine vinegar

2 Tbsp. fresh lemon juice

¾ cup low-sodium tomato juice

1 avocado, peeled and pitted, divided

½ teaspoon ground black pepper, divided

½ teaspoon sea salt, divided

1 lb. fresh bay scallops (tiny size)

2 Tbsp. extra virgin olive oil

In a blender, add tomatoes, cucumber, red pepper, celery, scallions, cilantro, parsley, vinegar, lemon juice, tomato juice, half of avocado, ¼ tsp. black pepper, and ¼ tsp. salt. Blend until reaches desired consistency. Chill covered, in refrigerator for at least 1 hour or overnight to let flavors meld.

Pat scallops dry and season with remaining ¼ tsp. black pepper and ¼ tsp. salt. Heat oil in a nonstick skillet over high heat. Add scallops and sear about 2 minutes per side (or to desired doneness), until scallops are no longer translucent.

Chop remaining half of avocado. To serve, divide gazpacho between 4 bowls and top with scallops and avocado slices.

SERVES

4

Spinach Salad

INGREDIENTS

½ lb fresh spinach leaves

1 hardboiled egg (organic), sliced

1 medium size tomato, diced

1 cucumber, sliced

1 clove garlic, minced

½ red onion, minced

1 lemon

2 Tbsp. olive oil

In a large bowl, combine spinach leaves, tomato, cucumber, onion, and egg.

In a small bowl whisk olive oil, fresh squeezed lemon juice, and garlic. Add to salad.

Warm Spinach Chicken Salad

INGREDIENTS

1 1b spinach

1 whole cooked chicken breast (organic), diced

2 Tbsp. olive oil

2 cloves garlic

Ground pepper to taste

1 large tomato, diced

Wash greens and remove stems. Shake out leaves but some water can remain.

Heat oil in deep pot over medium heat. Add garlic to cook, stir for about 30 seconds.

Add spinach and cover to cook 1-3 minutes until leaves begin to wilt.

Uncover and stir/toss leaves. Cover for 3-5 minutes or until leaves are completely wilted.

Remove spinach from heat and place in large bowl. Add chicken and tomatoes, and ground pepper to taste.

Pear and Toasted Walnut Salad

INGREDIENTS

1 ½ Tbsp. shallots, minced

2 Tbsp. extra-virgin olive oil

2 Tbsp. white wine vinegar

¼ tsp. Dijon mustard

¼ tsp. freshly ground black pepper

6 cups baby arugula leaves

2 pears, thinly sliced

¼ cup toasted walnuts, chopped

Combine first 6 ingredients in a large bowl; stir with a whisk. Add arugula and pears to bowl; toss to coat. Place about 1 ½ cups salad on each of 4 plates; sprinkle each serving with 1 Tbsp. walnuts.

SERVES 4

Pomegranate Kale Salad

INGREDIENTS

5 packed cups of kale, minced

¼ head of red cabbage, finely shredded

¼ cup pine nuts

½ cup pomegranate seeds

1 lemon

3 Tbsp. olive oil

Ground pepper to taste

In a large bowl add kale, cabbage, pine nuts, and pomegranate seeds

In a separate bowl, whisk fresh squeezed lemon juice and olive oil. Add ground pepper to taste.

Add dressing to salad and mix well

Artichoke Salad

INGREDIENTS

1 red bell pepper, sliced into thin strips

1 cucumber, sliced

1 head romaine lettuce, cut into wedges

3 artichoke hearts, cut into wedges

3 cloves garlic, minced

2 tsp olive oil

2 tsp Dijon mustard

1 Tbsp. white wine vinegar

Ground pepper to taste

In a small bowl, combine and mix garlic, vinegar, Dijon mustard, and olive oil. Add ground pepper to taste.

Combine red pepper, cucumber, lettuce, and artichokes. Drizzle with dressing before serving.

Pear Walnut Salad

INGREDIENTS

5 packed cups salad greens

3 Tbsp. chopped walnuts

2 large eggs, hardboiled and sliced

1 Bartlett Pear, cored and sliced

1 Tbsp. white wine vinegar

1 Tbsp. olive oil

1 tsp Dijon mustard

In a small bowl, whisk vinegar, olive oil, and Dijon mustard until smooth.

In a large bowl, combine salad greens, walnuts, hardboiled eggs, and pear slices. Drizzle dressing over top of salad and toss.

Avocado Walnut Salad

INGREDIENTS

1 head romaine lettuce, torn

3 Tbsp. olive oil

2 Tbsp. vinegar

1 tsp lemon juice

3 avocados, peeled and pitted and sliced

¼ cup walnuts, chopped

In a small bowl, whisk together olive oil and vinegar.

In a large bowl, combine all ingredients and toss well.

Chicken and Cabbage Salad

INGREDIENTS

2 chicken breasts

3 cups cabbage, finely chopped

1 can of corn

3 cups cherry tomatoes, halved

½ cup green onion, chopped

1 ripe avocado

½ cup water

1 lime

¼ cup cilantro

Ground pepper to taste

Cook chicken in pan on medium heat until cooked through

Diced cooked chicken into small bits.

In a blender, blend avocado, fresh lime juice, and cilantro until smooth. Add ground pepper to taste

In a bowl combine, cabbage, corn, tomatoes, onion, and chicken. Add avocado dressing and mix well.

Oriental Salad

INGREDIENTS

1 ¼ lb. chicken tenders

½ cup seasoned rice vinegar

¼ cup peeled fresh ginger, sliced, + 2 Tbsp. finely grated

2 Tbsp. + 1 ½ tsp. Braggs Amino Acid

1 ½ Tbsp. dark sesame oil

2 Tbsp. extra-virgin olive oil

¼ cup coarsely chopped scallions

1 small Napa cabbage, cut length-wise into thin slices

1 yellow bell pepper, cut into thin strips

1 large carrot, cut into thin strips

2 Tbsp. toasted sesame seeds

Rinse chicken and pat dry.

Bring 4 cups water, ¼ cup rice vinegar, ginger slices, and 2 Tbsp. Braggs Amino Acid to a boil in a large saucepan. Add chicken; simmer 1 minute. Remove pan from heat and let stand, covered, until chicken is cooked, about 5 minutes. Drain pan and discard ginger slices. Transfer chicken to a cutting board and slice.

To make dressing, whisk together remaining rice vinegar, the grated ginger, remaining soy sauce, sesame oil, olive oil, 2 Tbsp. water, and scallions in a large bowl; add salt and pepper to taste.

Toss cabbage, bell pepper, and carrot together. Top with chicken slices and sesame seeds and drizzle with dressing.

Avocado Egg Salad

INGREDIENTS

Hard boiled eggs (as many as you would like), diced

½ cup onion, diced

½ cup celery, diced

½ ripe avocado, mashed

1 Tbsp. Dijon mustard

1 tsp paprika

Ground pepper to taste

In a bowl combine eggs, onions, celery, avocado, and mustard. Stir well. Add paprika and pepper to taste before serving.

Grilled Salmon Salad

INGREDIENTS

½ cup olive oil

1 tsp. minced garlic

2 avocados, mashed

¼ cup chopped cilantro

¼ cup fresh lime juice

1 tomato, diced

3 salmon fillets

1 red onion, slice into rings

¼ cup extra virgin olive oil

1 head romaine lettuce,
remove exterior and hard
shell, chop remaining

In a bowl combine and whisk olive oil, lime juice, garlic and cilantro until well blended.

Add avocado and tomatoes and stir. Set aside.

Lightly coat salmon and onion rings with olive oil. Grill both until onion is brown and salmon is cooked through.

Place romaine in large bowl and add half of dressing. Top with salmon and onion rings.

Pour the remaining dressing over the top of the salmon and onions.

Avocado Fruit Salad

INGREDIENTS

1 grapefruit, halved

1 Tbsp. olive oil

1 Tbsp. basil, finely chopped

1 apple, cut julienne

2 radishes, thinly sliced

½ cup pomegranate arils

1 ripe avocado, cut in half and
remove pit and slice

In a small bowl, whisk fresh squeezed grapefruit juice, olive oil, and basil. Set bowl aside.

Gently toss apple, radishes, pomegranate arils, and avocado. Add grapefruit vinaigrette.

Not Your Average Chicken Salad

INGREDIENTS

3 cups cooked (organic) chicken, shredded

2 stalks celery, chopped

½ onion

2 Tbsp. olive oil

1 lemon, juiced

2 tsp. mustard

Ground pepper to taste

Add chicken, celery, and onion to a bowl.

Mix olive oil, lemon juice, and mustard and drizzle over top. Toss salad. Add pepper to taste.

Vitamin C Chicken

INGREDIENTS

¼ cup fresh orange juice

½ tsp. grated lime rind

2 Tbsp. fresh lime juice

2 Tbsp. fresh thyme, chopped

1 Tbsp. garlic, minced

1 tsp. grated orange rind

½ red pepper flakes

1 lb. skinless, boneless chicken breast cutlets

1 Tbsp. extra-virgin olive oil

½ cup fresh pineapple pieces

Olive oil cooking spray

6 cups bagged prewashed baby spinach

Combine first 8 ingredients in a small bowl, stirring well with a whisk. Pour ¼ cup juice mixture into a large Ziploc plastic bag. Add chicken to bag. Seal; let stand for 5 minutes. Add oil to remaining juice mixture; stir well with a whisk.

Heat a large nonstick skillet over medium-high heat. Coat the pan with cooking spray. Remove chicken from bag; discard marinade. Add chicken to pan along with pineapple pieces; cook 4 minutes on each side or until done. Place 1½ cups spinach on each of 4 plates. Divide chicken evenly among servings; top each serving with 1 Tbsp. juice mixture.

Chicken Marsala

INGREDIENTS

4 boneless, skinless chicken breasts

2 tsp. ground fennel seeds

1 tsp. red pepper flakes

16 small carrots, peeled

3 ½ cups Marsala wine

8 pieces dried porcini mushrooms

3 shallots, thinly sliced

2 tsp. garlic, smashed

Olive oil cooking spray

Garnish: sprigs of rosemary

Mix fennel, pepper, and red pepper flakes in a bowl. Sprinkle spice mix over chicken and set aside.

Place carrots in boiling water for about 4 minutes and remove. Dry on a paper towel. Set aside.

Bring Marsala or chicken broth to a low boil in a small saucepan over medium heat. Add mushrooms, shallots, and garlic. Simmer until sauce reduces, about 20 minutes. Discard garlic and set sauce aside.

Coat grill with cooking spray and grill chicken 4 to 6 minutes on each side or until cooked through.

Grill carrots about 5 minutes, rotating until charred. Return sauce to stove. Bring to a simmer, then remove from heat. Divide carrots among four plates and top with chicken, sauce, and a sprig of rosemary.

SERVES

4

Skillet Garlic Chicken

INGREDIENTS

2 chicken breasts (organic)

1 tsp onion powder

1 clove garlic, minced

2 Tbsp. olive oil

Ground pepper to taste

In a large skillet over medium heat, sauté garlic with 1 Tbsp. olive oil for about 2 minutes. Add 1 Tbsp. of olive oil and chicken; cook over medium-high heat for about 10-15 minutes on each side. Sprinkle onion powder and ground pepper over top while cooking.

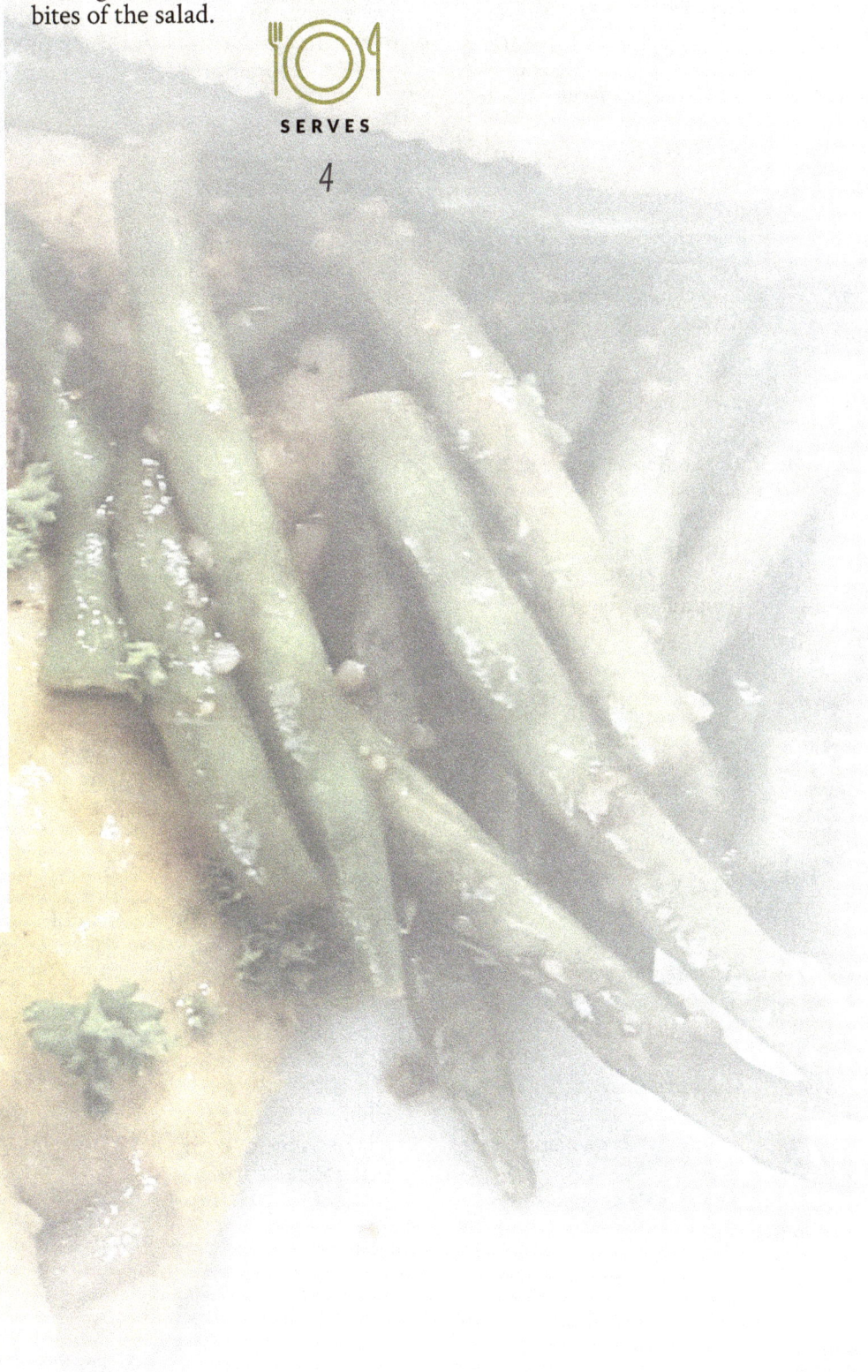

Yummy Tummy Chicken Chaat

INGREDIENTS

¾ cup Spanish onion, coarsely chopped

2 Tbsp. cilantro leaves, chopped

1 tsp. garlic, minced

1 Tbsp. extra-virgin olive oil

1 tsp. freshly squeezed lime juice + 4 lime halves for garnish

1 Tbsp. lemon juice

2 tsp. garam masala (available at specialty food stores and Indian markets)

1 tsp. hot green pepper, chopped

1 ½ tsp. red chili powder

½ tsp. red pepper flakes

1 lb. boneless, skinless chicken breasts, steamed, sliced lengthwise

8 iceberg lettuce leaves

Put the onion, cilantro, garlic, olive oil, lime and lemon juice, garam masala, green pepper, chili powder, and red pepper flakes in a large bowl and mix to create a sauce. Add the chicken and toss well. Divide the chicken among 4 small plates and serve with iceberg lettuce leaves and lime halves. Use the lettuce to scoop up bites of the salad.

SERVES

4

Parchment-Baked Herb Chicken

INGREDIENTS

2 sections of parchment paper, 12x16 inch pieces (one chicken breast per paper)

1 cup arugula leaves, divided

2 chicken breasts (organic), halved

1 tsp chopped sage, divided

1 tsp chopped rosemary, divided

1 cup chopped plum tomatoes, divided

1 cup onion, chopped and divided

2 tsp olive oil

Ground pepper to taste

Heat the oven to 450°

Fold parchment paper in half to create crease. Unfold paper and lightly coat with cooking spray in middle of paper.

Place ½ cup arugula on one side of parchment. Place chicken breast over arugula. Drizzle with 1 tsp olive oil, sprinkle with ½ tsp sage and ½ tsp rosemary. Add ½ cup tomatoes and ½ cup onions.

Fold parchment over chicken and seal edges with a fold.

Repeat with remaining parchment, herbs, chicken, tomato, and onion.

Place parchment packets on a baking sheet and bake for 20 minutes (should turn light brown). After baking, open packets and serve.

Spicy Mustard Chicken

INGREDIENTS

2 chicken breasts (organic)

1 tsp paprika

4 lemon slices

¼ cup spicy brown mustard

½ cup finely chopped onion

½ tsp lemon juice

½ tsp curry powder

Heat oven to 375°

Lightly coat a baking pan with olive oil. Arrange chicken breasts on pan. Sprinkle paprika over top of chicken. Place 2 lemon slices on each chicken breast. Bake for 20 minutes.

In a small sauce pan over low heat, combine mustard, onion, lemon juice, and curry powder. Mix well.

When chicken has cooked for 30 minutes, drain/discard juice. Drizzle sauce over top of chicken and baked for 15 more minutes or until cooked through.

Skillet Tomato Chicken

INGREDIENTS

2 chicken breasts (organic)

½ onion, finely chopped

½ green pepper, chopped

½ red bell pepper, chopped

1 qt no salt canned tomatoes

1 clove garlic, minced

2 tsp cumin

2 tsp chili powder

½ cup cilantro, finely chopped

1 Tbsp. olive oil

Ground pepper to taste

In large skillet, sauté chicken and olive oil until chicken is browned (about 4 minutes each side). Place chicken on a plate and cover to keep warm.

Add garlic, onion, and peppers to skillet, sauté for about 3 minutes. Add tomatoes with their juice to the skillet. Let the tomato juice come to a boil and then bring down to a simmer immediately following.

Add chicken back to skillet. Add cumin, chili powder, and cilantro. Cook for 5 minutes covered. Then, turn heat off and leave covered on stove-top for 5 more minutes. Add ground pepper to taste before serving.

Crockpot Salsa Chicken

INGREDIENTS

3-4 lbs chicken breast (organic)

4 large tomatoes, diced

½ onion, diced

1 lime, juiced

1 red bell pepper, diced

1 cup of your favorite salsa

2 Tbsp. red pepper flakes

1 tsp cayenne pepper

Ground pepper to taste

Combine all ingredients in crock-pot and cook on low for about 7 hours. After the chicken is cooked, shred in the crock-pot using a fork and knife. Mix well and let cool before serving.

Rosemary Chicken and Potatoes

INGREDIENTS

2 small red potatoes

2 small Yukon Gold potatoes

2 chicken breasts (organic)

½ red onion, chopped

½ cup celery, chopped

1 Tbsp. fresh rosemary, chopped

1 clove garlic, minced

Ground pepper to taste

1 lemon (juice)

1 Tbsp. olive oil

In medium saucepan, add potatoes and water (should cover potatoes). Bring water to a boil over high heat for about 15 minutes or until potatoes are tender. Drain and let potatoes cool before dicing.

In separate medium saucepan, poach chicken over medium-high heat for about 15-20 minutes or until they are no longer pink in the center. Drain and let cool before cutting chicken into small pieces.

In a large bowl combine all ingredients and mix well.

Turkey Loaf

INGREDIENTS

1 lb ground turkey

1 egg

2 large carrots, finely chopped

1 large onion, finely chopped

1 red bell pepper, diced

1 stalk celery, finely chopped

1 Tbsp. Worcestershire sauce

1 Tbsp. whole grain mustard

½ tsp garlic pepper powder

Preheat oven to 350°

Combine all ingredients. Put into loaf pan. Cook for 1 hour.

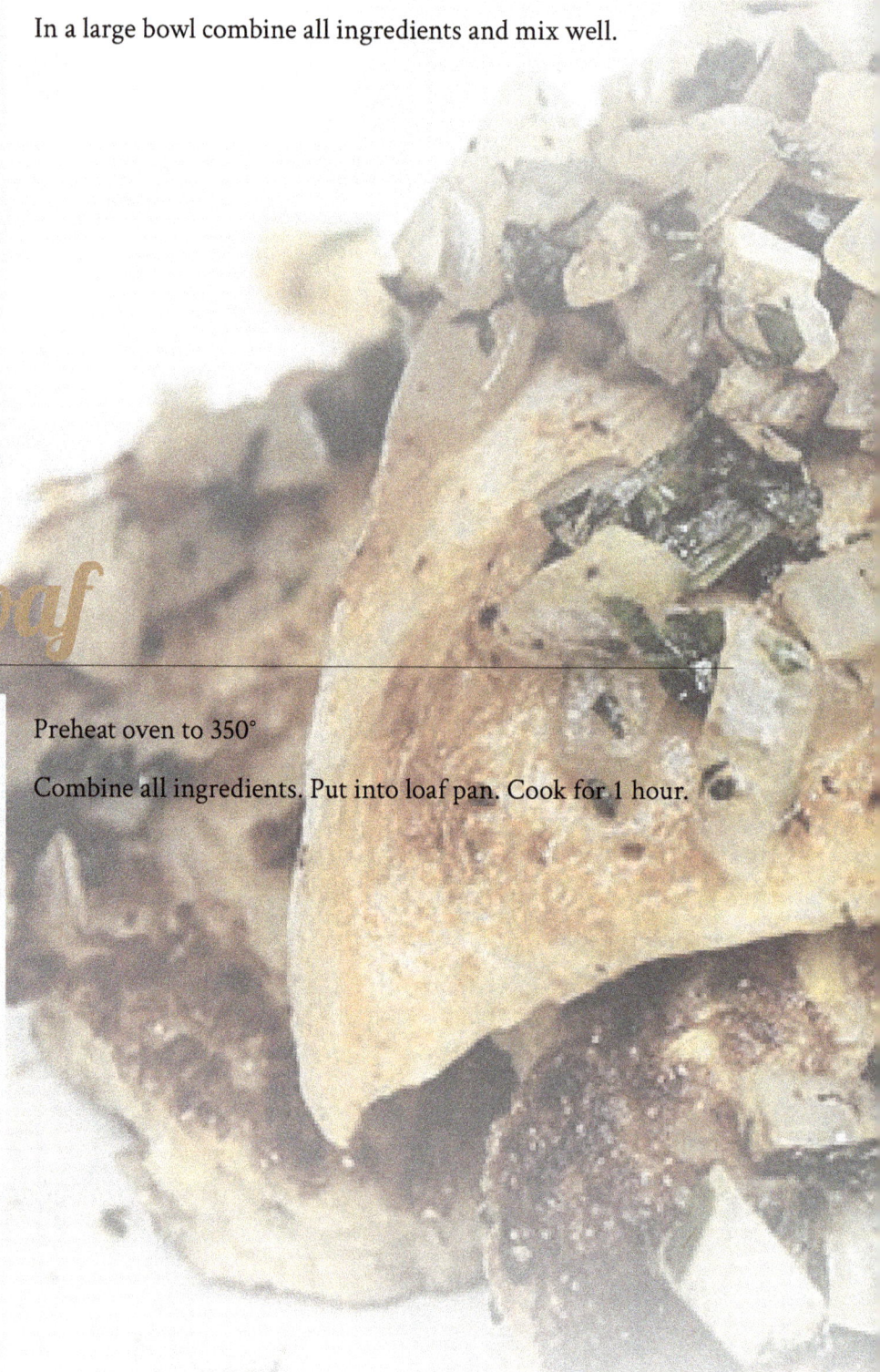

Mini Kale Turkey Burgers

INGREDIENTS

1 lb ground turkey

1 red onion, chopped

2 cups kale, finely chopped

2 cloves garlic, minced

1 egg

2 Tbsp. canola oil

1 tsp crushed chili pepper

1 tsp paprika

1 tsp cumin

Ground pepper to taste

In large bowl, mix ground turkey, onion, garlic, kale, egg, chili pepper, paprika, cumin and pepper.

Form mixture into mini burgers

Add canola oil to pan and cook burgers over medium heat for about 7 minutes each side.

Can serve with homemade marinara.

Pomegranate Pork

INGREDIENTS

½ tsp cinnamon

½ tsp cumin

1 tsp paprika

2 Tbsp. olive oil

2 pork tenderloins

1 cup 100% pomegranate juice

1 ½ cup pomegranate arils

2 tsp balsamic vinegar

Heat the oven to 350°F

In a medium bowl, combine the dry spices. Season tenderloins with mixture.

In large skillet, heat olive oil over medium-high heat for 1-2 minutes (should get hot but not smoky). Reduce heat, add pork and cook until browned all over. Transfer pork into baking dish or on baking sheet to bake for 20 minutes. Remove and transfer to cutting board, cover with foil and let sit for 10 minutes.

In a medium skillet over medium-high heat, add pomegranate juice and let come to a boil for 2-3 minutes. Remove from heat.

Drizzle juice, balsamic oil, and pomegranate arils over the top of the tenderloins before serving.

Guacamole Turkey Patties

INGREDIENTS

2 lb lean ground turkey

3 tsp ground cinnamon

1 tsp garlic powder

1 tsp ground black pepper

Guacamole Spread
Ingredients:

2 avocados, peeled and pitted

1 tsp garlic powder

½ tsp ground pepper

1 jalapeño, seeded and finely
chopped

½ onion, chopped

1 lime, juiced

In a large bowl, mix ground turkey, cinnamon, garlic powder, and ground pepper and form into flat patties.

Heat skillet or griddle to medium-high heat and cook patties 7-9 minutes on each side or until they are cooked through.

In a medium bowl combine avocado, garlic powder, ground pepper, jalapenos, onion, and lime juice. Mix ingredients to the consistency of your choice (chunky or smooth).

After patties are cooked, spread Guacamole over top of patties before serving (DO NOT use a bun if in PHASE 1. Could serve in lettuce wrap.)

Tasty Tuna Salad

INGREDIENTS

1 can solid white tuna,
drained

8 cherry tomatoes

½ onion, chopped

½ small head of lettuce, torn

1 stalk celery, chopped

½ green pepper, chopped

2 Tbsp. olive oil

¼ tsp. garlic powder

Shred tuna. Combine all ingredients and let marinate in refrigerator for 1 hour before serving.

Eggplant Tuna Salad

INGREDIENTS

1 eggplant, peeled and cubed

2 tsp olive oil, divided

1 6oz can tuna in water, drained

2 stalks celery, chopped

1 cup chopped onion

1 Tbsp. vinegar

½ tsp Dijon mustard

In medium skillet over medium heat, sauté eggplant with 1 tsp olive oil for about 5 minutes. Let cool.

In a small bowl, whisk 1 tsp olive oil, vinegar and mustard.

In a medium bowl, combine tuna, celery, onion, and cooled eggplant. Add dressing and lightly toss before serving.

Walnut Crusted Salmon

INGREDIENTS

1 lb salmon fillets

1 cup crushed/ground walnuts

½ tsp ground coriander

½ tsp ground cumin

1 lemon, juiced

1 tsp coconut oil

Ground pepper to taste

Heat oven to 350°

Drizzle lemon juice over salmon fillets. And season with ground pepper.

In a medium bowl, combine ground crushed walnuts, coriander, and cumin. Dip fillets into mixture and evenly coat on both sides.

Lightly grease broiler pan with coconut oil. Place fillets on pan and bake for 12-15 minutes.

Lemon Salmon with Avocado Salsa

INGREDIENTS

Salmon Ingredients:

2 (5-oz) salmon filets

2 tsp olive oil

½ lemon (grate peel)

1 tsp fennel seeds

1 tsp mustard seeds

Ground pepper to taste

Avocado Salsa Ingredients:

½ lemon (juice)

1 avocado, chopped

2 Roma tomatoes, chopped

1 Tbsp. olive oil

1 onion, finely chopped

Ground pepper to taste

Heat oven to 450°

Place salmon on sheet of foil. Drizzle olive oil over top of salmon. Sprinkle lemon zest and seeds over the top of salmon. Add pepper to taste.

Bake for 10-12 minutes.

Prepare avocado salsa in small bowl. Chop avocado, tomatoes, and onion. Drizzle lemon juice and olive oil. Add pepper to taste.

Add salsa to the top of the salmon before serving.

Asian Salmon Marinade

INGREDIENTS

2 lbs. salmon

2 Tbsp. Dijon mustard

3 Tbsp. Braggs Amino Acid or tamari sauce

4 Tbsp. extra-virgin olive oil

2 tsp. garlic, minced

Marinade salmon in refrigerator for 1 hour.

Then cook salmon until pink in the middle at 400 degrees for about 15 minutes.

Cilantro Ginger Baked Tilapia

INGREDIENTS

1 lb tilapia fillets

Ground pepper

3 cloves garlic, peeled and mashed

1 Tbsp. grated fresh ginger

1 jalapeno, seeded and chopped

1/3 cup chopped cilantro leaves

1 lemon, juiced

2 Tbsp. low sodium soy sauce

1 tsp sesame oil

Heat oven to 450°.

Season fillets with ground pepper and lay flat in 9x9 glass baking dish.

In a blender, blend garlic, ginger, jalapeno, cilantro, lemon juice, soy sauce, and sesame oil. Pour sauce over fillets.

Bake fillets for about 30 minutes.

Sautéed Shrimp and Broccoli

INGREDIENTS

20 large shrimp peeled

2 gloves garlic, minced

1 ½ lbs broccoli, cut into small florets

1 lime

3 tsp olive oil, reserve 1 tsp for sauté

1 tsp ginger

1 tsp red chili flakes

In a bowl mix garlic, ginger, fresh lime juice, and olive oil with shrimp. Let it marinate for a few minutes in the refrigerator while preparing broccoli.

Steam broccoli for 5 minutes in vegetable steamer

Sauté shrimp in reserved olive oil in large pan for 5 minutes or until the shrimp turns pink. Add broccoli and cook for additional 5 minutes.

Sprinkle red chili flakes over top before serving

Fresh Veggie Ceviche

INGREDIENTS

1 lb bay scallops or 1 lb halibut fillets or 1 lb sea bass fillets, or 1 lb jumbo shrimp or a mixture of fish

8 limes, juiced

2 large tomatoes, diced

4 green onions, minced

2 stalks celery, chopped

1 bell pepper, chopped

½ cup chopped parsley

1 ½ Tbsp. olive oil

1/8 cup chopped cilantro

Ground pepper to taste

Rinse scallops and place in medium bowl. Pour lime juice over top so scallops are completely immersed in juice. Let chill all day or overnight until scallops turn opaque. Empty half of lime juice from bowl.

Add remaining ingredients and stir gently.

Garlic Roasted Shrimp

INGREDIENTS

¼ cup olive oil

5 sprigs rosemary

3 cloves garlic, minced

½ cup chopped onion

2 lbs shrimp, peeled and deveined

2 Tbsp. white wine vinegar

½ tsp ground pepper

Pour olive oil into 9x13 inch baking dish/roasting pan. Add rosemary, garlic, and onion and let dish sit in oven as it preheats to 450° (about 15 minutes). Remove pan.

Add shrimp over the top and roast until pink and firm (8 minutes for medium shrimp, 10 minutes for large shrimp). Gently toss halfway through baking.

Remove dish from oven and add vinegar and ground pepper. Stir gently before serving.

Avocado Shrimp

INGREDIENTS

1 lb jumbo shrimp, peeled and deveined

1 medium tomato, diced

1 avocado, peeled and pitted and diced

½ jalapeno, seeded and chopped

¼ cup chopped red bell pepper, seeded

¼ cup finely chopped onion

2 limes, juiced

1 tsp olive oil

1 Tbsp. chopped cilantro

Ground pepper to taste

In a small bowl, combine onion, lime juice, olive oil, and ground pepper and let marinate for about 5 minutes.

Combine remaining ingredients.

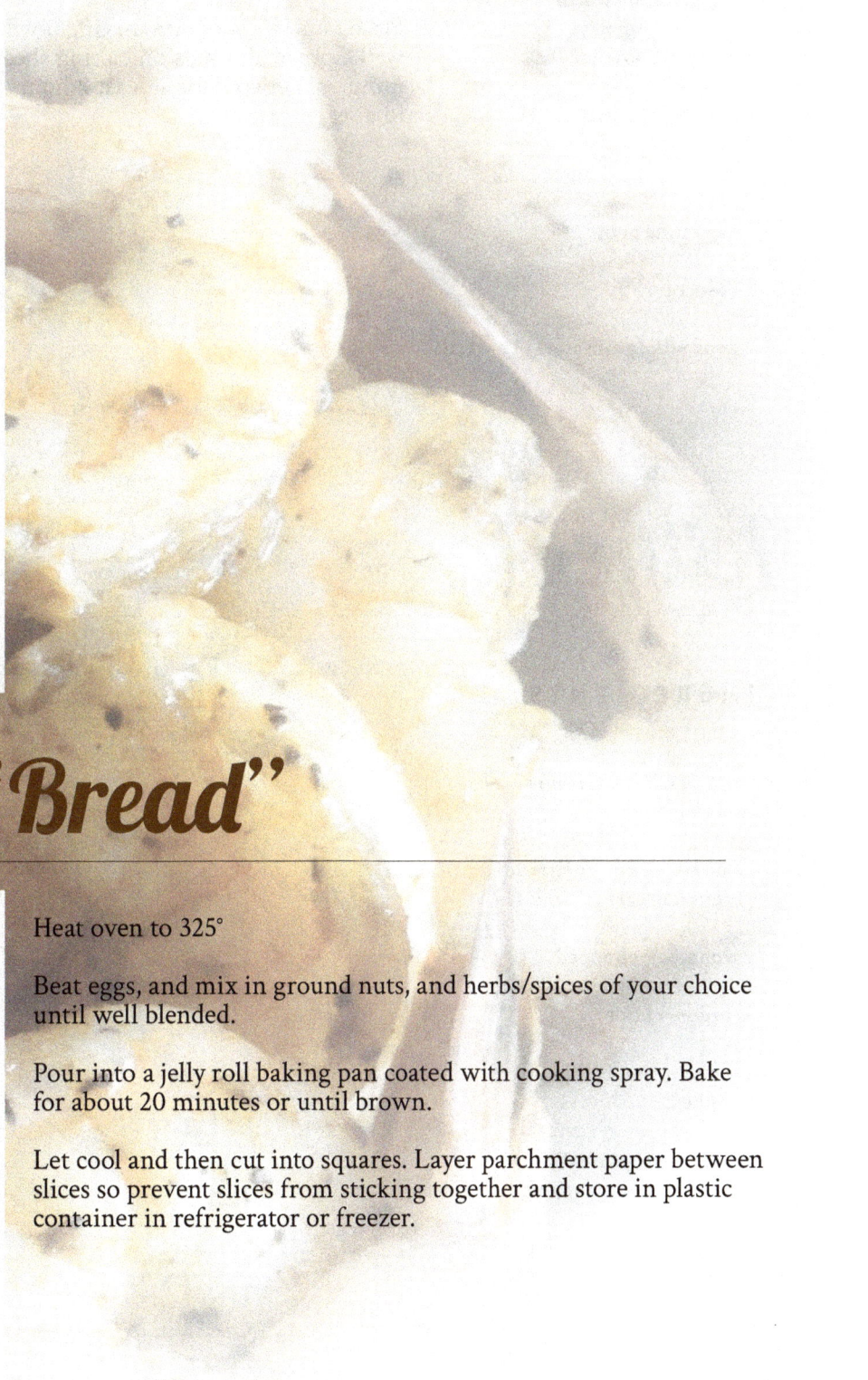

Protein "Bread"

INGREDIENTS

7 eggs (organic)- all egg whites for lighter bread and whole eggs for heavier bread

½ lb nuts of choice (almonds or pecans recommended), chopped and ground

Add your favorite herbs/ spices

Heat oven to 325°

Beat eggs, and mix in ground nuts, and herbs/spices of your choice until well blended.

Pour into a jelly roll baking pan coated with cooking spray. Bake for about 20 minutes or until brown.

Let cool and then cut into squares. Layer parchment paper between slices so prevent slices from sticking together and store in plastic container in refrigerator or freezer.

Spiced Almonds

INGREDIENTS

½ tsp ground cumin

½ tsp chili powder

½ tsp garlic powder

¼ tsp cayenne pepper

¼ tsp cinnamon

1 Tbsp. olive oil

2 cups whole almonds

Heat oven to 325°

In a small nonstick skillet over low heat, mix all ingredients except for almonds. Let simmer for about 2-4 minutes.

Place nuts in a medium mixing bowl and add spice mixture, mix well. Spread almonds on baking sheet and bake for about 15 minutes. Let cool for at least 2 hours before serving. Can be stored in a sealed jar.

Lettuce tacos

INGREDIENTS

Romaine lettuce leaves (whole)

Ground turkey or shredded chicken breast

2 tomatoes, chopped

½ onion, chopped

1 red or green bell pepper, chopped

1 jalapeno (optional), de-seeded and chopped

1 Tbsp. fresh lime juice

Cook ground turkey in skillet. Mix all ingredients and at lime juice.

Wrap ingredients in lettuce

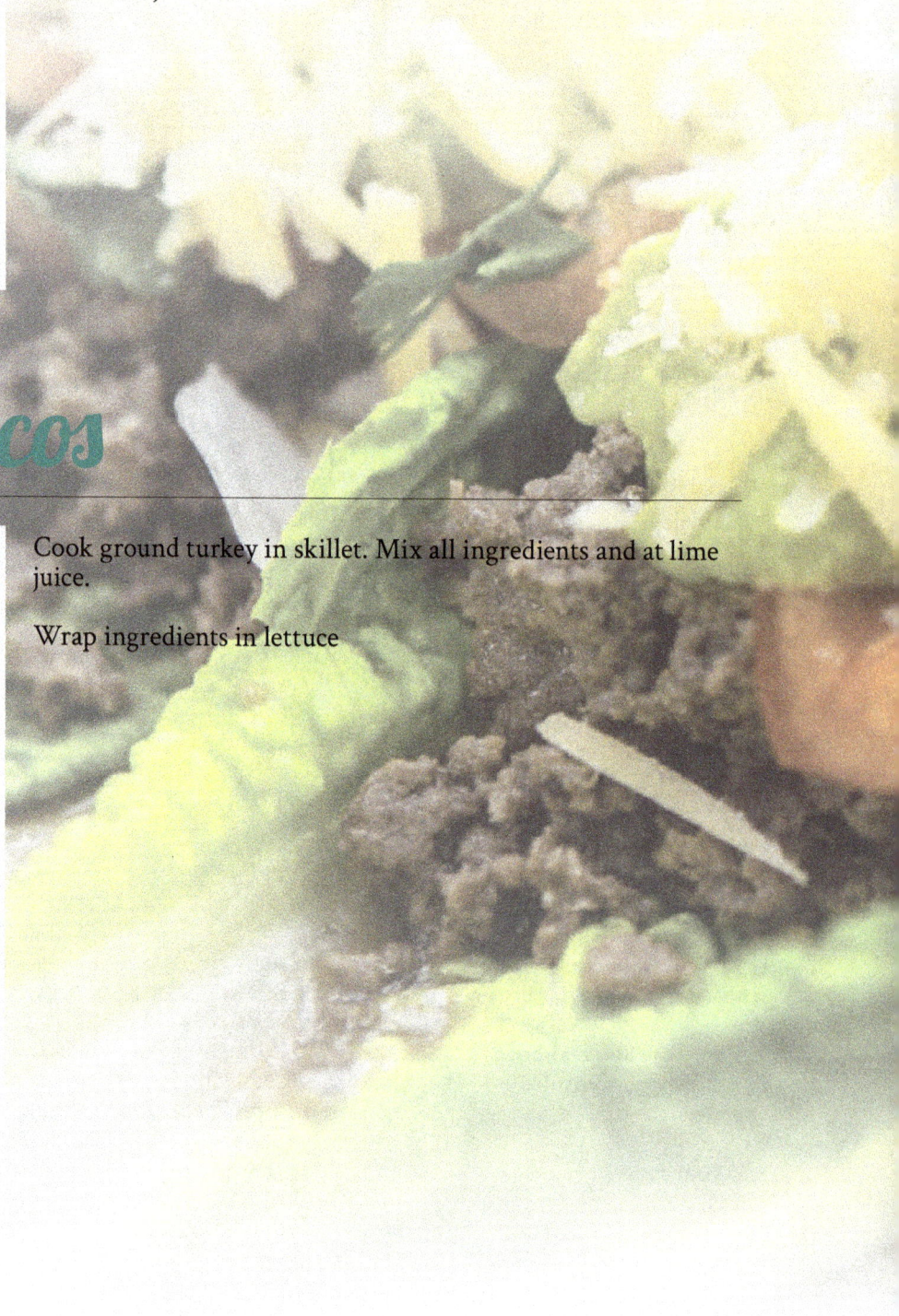

Avocado Spicy Shrimp Lettuce Wraps

INGREDIENTS

Spicy Shrimp Ingredients:

15-20 shrimp, peeled and deveined

½ tsp paprika

½ tsp cumin

½ tsp hot chili powder

½ tsp Ground pepper

½ Tbsp. olive oil

½ lime, juiced

1 scallion, chopped

½ cup baby arugula

2 Roma tomatoes, diced

1 head Romaine lettuce (leave whole)

Jalapeño Avocado Sauce Ingredients:

1 avocado

1 clove garlic

1 jalapeño, seeded and chopped

½ lime, juiced

1 Tbsp. chopped cilantro

In a large bowl combine shrimp, paprika, cumin, chili powder, and ground pepper.

In a skillet, sauté shrimp in olive oil on medium heat for about 3 minutes (shrimp should turn pink). Squeezed ½ lime over top of shrimp while cooking.

In a blender combine all sauce ingredients and blend until smooth.

On a large lettuce leaf, place arugula, shrimp, scallions, tomato and sauce.

Nutrient Rich Food to Incorporate into Your Routine:

Avocados

Chard, collard greens, kale, mustard greens, spinach

Bell peppers

Brussels sprouts

Mushrooms (crimini and shiitake)

Baked potatoes

Sweet potatoes

Cantaloupe, papaya, raspberries, strawberries

Low-fat yogurt

Eggs

Seeds (flax, pumpkin, sesame, and sunflower)

Dried beans (garbanzo, kidney, navy, pinto)

Lentils, peas

Almonds, cashews, peanuts

Barley, oats, quinoa, brown rice

Salmon, halibut, cod, scallops, shrimp, tuna

Lean beef, lamb, venison

Chicken, turkey

Almond Flax Pizza Crust

INGREDIENTS

1-1/4 cups flaxseed meal

1 cup almond flour/meal

1 tsp sea salt

2 tsp natural baking powder

1 Tbsp. honey

1 tsp Italian mixed dried herbs

3 large eggs, beaten until smooth

3 Tbsp. coconut oil, melted

½ cup water

Heat oven to 425° F.

Combine flaxseed meal, almond meal, sea salt, baking powder and Italian herbs together until lump-free.

Beat together eggs, oil, honey and water until smooth.

Pour liquid mixture into dry mixture. Blend well until smooth.

Press into desired shape.

Place on a pre-greased or non-stick pizza pan or sit on a silicon baking mat.

Bake for 15 minutes in the center of the oven until cooked.

Add favorite toppings and then return to the oven to bake for an additional 10-15 minutes.

Top with olive oil, homemade tomato sauce, and fresh vegetables

SERVES

4

Tasty Tomato Sauce

INGREDIENTS

8 medium Roma tomatoes

1 Tbsp. extra-virgin olive oil

1 white onion, diced

1 ½ Tbsp. garlic, chopped

2 Tbsp. tomato paste

8 large basil leaves

2 tsp. raw organic honey or Stevia

Bring a pot of water to boil over high heat. While water is boiling, use a small knife to remove each tomato core and cut a tiny X into the bottom of each tomato.

Prepare an ice bath in a large bowl. Immerse tomatoes into boiling water for 1 to 2 minutes or until skin begins to come off. Remove tomatoes with a slotted spoon and immerse into ice baht for about 1 minute or until cooled. Once cooked, remove tomatoes from water and remove skin by peeling it back from the X in the bottom. Slice tomatoes in half, scoop out and discard seeds. Coarsely chop tomatoes and place into a bowl.

In a medium saucepot, heat oil over medium-high heat. Add onion and garlic and sauté until onion becomes translucent. Add tomatoes, tomato paste, and basil and cook, stirring frequently, until sauce comes to a boil. Reduce heat to medium-low and simmer for 45 minutes to 1 hour, stirring frequently.

Remove from heat and puree with a hand blender until smooth. Add honey/Stevia and mix well.

Ladle sauce into re-sealable containers, let cool to room temperature, cover and refrigerate until needed. Sauce can be kept refrigerated for up to 5 days or frozen for up to 2 months.

Guacamole

INGREDIENTS

3 ripe avocadoes

Juice of ½ fresh lime

2 Tbsp. chopped cilantro

½ red or purple onion, minced well

1 tsp. garlic, minced

1 jalapeno, chopped

Cut avocados in half. Discard pit and scoop flesh into bowl. Place all ingredients in medium bowl and mix until just combined. Don't over mix.

SERVES

6

Pico de Gallo

INGREDIENTS

4-6 Roma tomatoes

1 red bell pepper

1 jalapeño (optional)

½ onion

1 lime

1 clove garlic, minced

Cilantro

Ground pepper to taste

Cut tomatoes, red pepper, onion, and garlic into small pieces, may discard seeds (of tomato and red pepper) if desired. Combine in a bowl

Cut stems off cilantro. Chop leaves and add to bowl.

De-seed jalapeno and cut to small pieces. Only add as much pepper as wanted for spice. (Whole pepper or more=spicy, half or less=mild)

Add fresh squeezed lime juice to taste. Add ground pepper to taste.

Avocado Salsa

INGREDIENTS

½ lemon (juice)

1 avocado, peeled and pitted and chopped

2 Roma tomatoes, chopped

1 Tbsp. olive oil

1 onion, finely chopped

1 clove garlic, minced

Ground pepper to taste

Combine all ingredients and toss well.

Mango Pepper Salsa

INGREDIENTS

4 red bell peppers, chopped

2 large ripe mangos, diced

2 scallions, sliced

1 jalapeno

½ lime (juice)

1 bunch cilantro, finely chopped

Combine all ingredients and toss well.

Granny Apple Vinaigrette

INGREDIENTS

½ cup walnut oil

¼ cup apple cider vinegar

1 Gala apple, peeled, cored, and cut into small pieces

½ tsp. paprika

½ tsp. cinnamon

½ tsp. red pepper flakes

Add all ingredients to a blender or mini food processor and puree until everything is finely diced. Add to your favorite salad.

Pesto Vinaigrette Salad

INGREDIENTS

1 medium ripe tomato, cored and chopped (about 1 cup)

1 cup jarred artichoke hearts packed in water, drained, rinsed, and quartered

5-6 ounces baby arugula (about 5 ½ cups lightly packed)

2 Tbsp. red wine vinegar

2 Tbsp. basil pesto

Arrange the tomato and artichoke hearts over a bed of arugula. Whisk together the vinegar and pesto, drizzle over the salad, and serve.

Red Wine Vinaigrette

INGREDIENTS

2 cloves garlic, minced

2 Tbsp. Dijon mustard

½ cup red wine vinegar

1 tsp ground pepper

1 cup olive oil

½ cup chopped basil leaves

½ cup chopped parsley

Combine and whisk all ingredients.

Shallot Vinaigrette

Combine and whisk all ingredients

INGREDIENTS

2 Tbsp. red wine vinegar

1 Tbsp. Dijon mustard

¼ cup olive oil

1 Tbsp. finely chopped shallots

Ground pepper to taste

Caesar Dressing

INGREDIENTS

1 clove garlic, minced

1 tsp dry mustard

1 Tbsp. lemon juice

1 tsp cayenne pepper

2 Tbsp. olive oil

Ground pepper to taste

In a small bowl, whisk garlic, dry mustard, lemon juice, cayenne pepper, and olive oil. Add ground pepper to taste.

Garlic Dressing

INGREDIENTS

½ tsp dry mustard

1 tsp ground pepper

2 cloves garlic, finely minced

1 Tbsp. tarragon vinegar

2 Tbsp. lemon juice

3 Tbsp. olive oil

Combine all ingredients and mix well.

Ginger-Soy Salad Dressing

INGREDIENTS

1 Tbsp. fresh ginger, minced

2 Tbsp. Braggs Amino Acid or tamari sauce

2 ½ Tbsp. rice wine vinegar

½ cup sesame oil

¼ cup extra-virgin olive oil

Mix all the ingredients together and put on salad or marinade meat of your choice.

Wasabi Dressing

INGREDIENTS

4 Tbsp. rice vinegar

2 Tbsp. extra-virgin olive oil

1 tsp. wasabi paste

1 tsp. pure sesame oil

½ tsp. toasted unsalted sesame seeds

In a small mixing bowl, whisk together all ingredients until blended. Refrigerate until serving or use immediately. Oil-based dressings last longest in the refrigerator (up to 2 weeks) but should be brought to room temperature before using for best flavor.

Low-Calorie Lemon Dressing

INGREDIENTS

6 oz. soft tofu, drained

2 Tbsp. fresh lemon juice

2 tsp. lemon zest

1 Tbsp. rice vinegar

1 Tbsp. extra-virgin olive oil

Sea salt and fresh ground black pepper, to taste

2 tsp. chives, chopped

Place tofu in a blender and process with lemon juice and zest, vinegar, and oil. Scrape down sides of work bowl as needed.

Transfer dressing to a small mixing or serving bowl and stir in salt, pepper, and chives. Refrigerate until serving or use immediately. Store in a sealed container in refrigerator for 1 to 2 days (dependent on shelf life of tofu).

Basil Nut Vinaigrette

INGREDIENTS

20 fresh basil leaves, finely chopped

1 tsp. garlic, minced

2 tsp. Dijon mustard

2 Tbsp. wine vinegar

2 Tbsp. extra-virgin olive oil

4 Tbsp. low-sodium chicken broth

Fresh ground black pepper, to taste

2 Tbsp. unsalted walnuts, chopped

In a medium-size mixing bowl, add basil, garlic, Dijon, vinegar, oil, broth, and pepper, whisking to combine thoroughly. Stir in walnuts. Refrigerate until serving or use immediately. Store in a sealed container in refrigerator for up to 2 weeks.

Mustard Dressing

INGREDIENTS

6 oz. soft tofu, drained

2 Tbsp. Dijon mustard

1 Tbsp. fresh lemon juice

2 tsp. garlic, chopped

1 tsp. dried tarragon

Place tofu in a blender and process with Dijon, lemon juice, and garlic until smooth, scraping down sides of work bowl as needed.

Transfer dressing to a small mixing or serving bowl and stir in tarragon. Refrigerate until serving or use immediately. Store in a sealed container in refrigerator for up to 3 days (dependent on shelf life of tofu).

Tomato Salad

INGREDIENTS

1 lb Roma tomatoes, cut into wedges

½ lb yellow cherry tomatoes, halved

½ lb red cherry tomatoes, halved

½ red onion, chopped

½ cup basil leaves

¼ cup olive oil

2 Tbsp. vinegar

In a bowl, combine all tomatoes, onion, basil, oil and vinegar and toss well.

Tomato and Cucumber salad

INGREDIENTS

1 cucumber

15-20 cherry tomatoes

½ onion, chopped

3 basil leaves, chopped

3 Tbsp. Olive oil

2 Tbsp. Vinegar

Ground black pepper to taste

Cut tomatoes in half. Cut cucumber (peeling optional) into slices and then into ¼.

Add onion and basil.

Mix oil and vinegar and drizzle over salad. Add pepper to taste.

Tomato Avocado Tartar

INGREDIENTS

1 lb asparagus, discard stem and chop remaining

1 lb cherry tomatoes, quartered

2 ripe avocados, peeled and cubed

2 Tbsp. olive oil

1 lemon

1 lime

1 oz tarragon, chopped

1 tsp agave

Ground pepper to taste

Steam asparagus 5-7 minutes

In a bowl combine tomatoes, avocado, asparagus and fresh squeezed lemon juice.

In a small bowl mix tarragon, olive oil, lime juice, agave, and ground pepper to taste.

Add dressing to vegetables and mix well.

Warm Veggie Salad

INGREDIENTS

1 green pepper, sliced

1 small cauliflower head, cut into florets

½ lb green beans, trimmed

1 pint cherry tomatoes

7 basil leaves, finely chopped

1 tsp. Dijon mustard

1 Tbsp. olive oil

Heat oven to 350°F

Blanch pepper, cauliflower and beans in boiling water for 3 minutes, drain water, place in oven dish and top with tomatoes

Combine olive oil, basil, and mustard. Drizzle over vegetables.

Bake for 10 minutes

Almond Broccoli Salad

INGREDIENTS

½ lb baby broccoli

1 Tbsp. olive oil

1 lemon, zest and juice

1 tsp ground black pepper

2 Tbsp. almonds, sliced

Heat oven to 400°. Line baking sheet with parchment paper. Arrange broccoli in rows on pan. Add almonds to free spaces on sheet. Drizzle olive oil, lemon zest, and lemon juice over the top. Bake for about 10-15 minutes or until broccoli stems are tender. Toss mixture before serving.

Roasted Florets and Peppers

INGREDIENTS

1 head broccoli florets

1 head cauliflower florets

1 red bell pepper, sliced

1 green bell pepper, sliced

1 orange or yellow bell pepper, sliced

½ onion, chopped

3 Tbsp. olive oil

¾ tsp red pepper flakes

Ground pepper to taste

Heat oven to 400°

Place all vegetables on a rimmed cookie sheet. Drizzle olive oil, red pepper flakes and ground pepper over top of vegetables. Roast for about 10 minutes and then flip vegetables over and roast another 10 minutes or until browned.

Lemon Roasted Peppers

INGREDIENTS

2 red bell peppers, seeded and sliced

2 green bell peppers, seeded and sliced

1 yellow bell pepper, seeded and sliced

1 orange bell pepper, seeded and sliced

5 small sweet peppers (any color), seeded and chopped

½ tsp olive oil

1 lemon, juiced

Ground pepper to taste

Set oven to broil

Place peppers on a baking sheet. Drizzle olive oil over top. Broil for 2-3 minutes or until skin is browned/blackened. Drizzle lemon juice over and ground pepper over top before serving.

Crispy Kale Chips

INGREDIENTS

4 cups kale, chopped

1 Tbsp. olive oil

¼ cup almonds, sliced

Seasoning of your choice
(paprika, garlic powder,
ground pepper, rosemary)

Heat oven to 275°.

In a medium bowl, toss kale leaves with olive oil, almonds, and seasoning. Lay mixture flat on a baking sheet. Bake for about 15-20 minutes (or until leaves are crispy), turning leaves halfway through.

Sweet and Spicy Apples and Potatoes

INGREDIENTS

2 sweet potatoes, peeled and diced

3 Tbsp. olive oil

½ firm apple (Granny Smith or honey crisp recommended), peeled/cored and diced

1 lemon (juice)

1 red chili pepper, stemmed/seeded and chopped

1 tsp chili flakes

Heat oven to 350°F

Place diced sweet potatoes in medium bowl and toss with 3 Tbsp. olive oil. Place potatoes on rimmed cookie sheet and cover with foil. Bake for about 20-25 minutes or until soft.

In a large skillet on low/medium heat, add the baked sweet potatoes. With a spatula, turn potatoes and cook until brown. Add apple, lemon juice, and chili pepper. Continue to cook until apples are warm. Sprinkle chili flakes over the top before serving.

Sweet Potato Fries

INGREDIENTS

3 sweet potatoes, sliced in strips

1 Tbsp. olive oil

1 tsp rosemary leaves, finely chopped

Ground pepper to taste

Heat oven to 425°F

In large bowl, toss sweet potatoes, rosemary, and olive oil until evenly coated. Place potatoes on parchment lined baking sheet. Bake for about 15 minutes, then flip potatoes and continue baking for about 15 more minutes or until lightly browned. Remove from oven and add pepper to taste before serving.

Sweet Potato Treat

INGREDIENTS

2 sweet potatoes (about 2 lbs. total), peeled and cut into ½-by-2-inch sticks

2 Tbsp. extra virgin olive oil

Sea salt and ground pepper

1 Tbsp. fresh lemon juice

1 Tbsp. cinnamon

Preheat oven to 450 degrees. Divide potatoes between two rimmed baking sheets; toss with oil, and season with salt and pepper. Arrange in a single layer, without overlapping. Roast, tossing once, until tender and starting to brown, 25 to 30 minutes.

Sprinkle with lemon juice and cinnamon; season with salt and pepper, if desired. Toss to coat.

PHASE 2

DURING PHASE 2, YOU WILL INTRODUCE SOME WHOLE GRAIN CHOICES AND MORE PROTEIN OPTIONS SUCH AS WHOLE EGGS, LEGUMES, BEANS, AND COTTAGE CHEESE BACK INTO YOUR EATING. IN GENERAL, AVOIDING DAIRY, ESPECIALLY MILK PRODUCTS AND CHEESE, WILL CONTINUE TO HELP WITH YOUR SUCCESS AND GOAL ATTAINMENT. BUY ORGANIC IF POSSIBLE. IF YOU DO CHOOSE TO ADD DAIRY BACK INTO YOUR EATING PLAN, PHASE IT IN SEPARATELY FROM THE GRAINS. YOUR MEAL SCHEDULE AND FREQUENCY SHOULD REMAIN THE SAME, BUT YOU NOW WILL HAVE A WIDER VARIETY OF FOODS TO CHOOSE FROM.

WHEN INTRODUCING FOODS BACK INTO YOUR PLAN, BE AWARE OF HOW THEY MAKE YOU FEEL. IF YOU PUT DAIRY OR ANY OTHER FOOD BACK INTO YOUR PLAN AND YOU FEEL SLUGGISH, HAVE DIGESTIVE ISSUES, OR ANY OTHER SYMPTOMS THAT WERE NOT PRESENT DURING PHASE 1, YOU MAY HAVE AN INTOLERANCE TO THAT PARTICULAR FOOD. IF THIS IS THE CASE, IT IS BEST TO AVOID THAT FOOD GROUP.

IN PHASE 2, THE MAJORITY OF CARBOHYDRATES WILL STILL COME FROM FRUITS AND VEGETABLES TO OBTAIN NEEDED NUTRITION, BUT YOU CAN ADD BACK ONE SERVING OF THE FOLLOWING GRAIN FOODS FOR BREAKFAST OR LUNCH:

• QUINOA • PEARLED BARLEY • BULGAR • BROWN RICE

• STEEL CUT OATS (NOTHING INSTANT) • WHOLE WHEAT/GRAIN BREADS OR PASTA

IF YOU ARE NOT LOSING WEIGHT AT ACCEPTABLE RATE, STOP THIS ADDITIONAL FOOD FIRST.

BREADS, PASTAS, ETC. MUST BE WHOLE GRAIN (EZEKIEL BREAD, WHICH IS SPROUTED GRAINS, IS THE BEST TYPE). IF YOU ARE WORKING OUT, YOU CAN ADD AN ADDITIONAL WHOLE GRAIN BREAD OR PASTA SERVING PRIOR TO A WORKOUT. ADD ONLY IF YOU NEED THE ENERGY TO DO AN EFFECTIVE WORKOUT, OTHERWISE EAT A SERVING OF FRUIT. REMEMBER A SERVING OF BREAD IS ONE SLICE AND A SERVING OF PASTA IS ½ CUP.

YOU CAN ALSO HAVE ONE SERVING OF THE FOLLOWING INSTEAD OF A BREAD OR PASTA:

• LEGUMES (BEANS/PEANUTS/PEAS) • STARCHY VEGGIES

AS FOR PROTEIN SOURCES, YOU CAN ADD BACK THE FOLLOWING:

• PLAIN GREEK YOGURT-MIX FRUIT IF NEEDED • COTTAGE CHEESE (1%-2% FAT)

• WHOLE EGGS (ORGANIC VS. FREE RANGE)-1 A DAY

YOU CAN ALSO ADD RICE OR ALMOND MILK (1 SERVING) INTO YOUR DAILY INTAKE IF DESIRED BUT THESE ARE GENERALLY A LOT LOWER IN PROTEIN THAN COW'S MILK.

WEST CLINIC 4 LIFE PHASE 2:
1 MONTH OF EASY EATING WEEK 1

Sunday	Monday	Tuesday	Wednesday	Thursday	Friday	Saturday
Meal 1 Protein loaded pancakes (pg 70)	Meal 1 Smoothie (pg 19-20, 76-78)	Meal 1 Greek yogurt, vanilla whey with fruit	Meal 1 Egg white omelet with vegetables	Meal 1 Oatmeal (pg 67-68) Fruit	Meal 1 100% Whole Wheat bread with natural peanut butter 1 Hard Boiled Egg	Meal 1 Christine's Frittata (pg 75)
Meal 2 Celery with natural peanut butter	Meal 2 ½ avocado with cottage cheese	Meal 2 2 Hard-boiled Eggs	Meal 2 Apple with natural peanut butter	Meal 2 Almonds Vegetable	Meal 2 Avocado Fruit Salad (pg 32)	Meal 2 Cottage cheese with tomato
Meal 3 Spinach Salad (pg 27) Cottage cheese	Meal 3 Warm Veggie Salad (pg 58)	Meal 3 Leftover Mini Kale Burgers (no bun) with Tasty Tomato Sauce (pg 48)	Meal 3 Lettuce wrap (pg 133-134)	Meal 3 Tuna (pg 142) Wrap	Meal 3 Homemade pizza (pg 139-157)	Meal 3 Summer vegetable medley (pg 212)
Meal 4 Lemon Chicken (pg 110)	Meal 4 Vegetable Almonds	Meal 4 Tomato Cucumber Salad (pg 57)	Meal 4 Pomegranate Kale Salad (pg 28)	Meal 4 Hard-boiled egg	Meal 4 Protein Shake	Meal 4 Leftover pizza
Meal 5 Vegetable	Meal 5 Mini Kale Burgers (pg 39) on whole wheat bun	Meal 5 JR's Power Salad (pg 94)	Meal 5 Carrots with hummus	Meal 5 Cottage cheese with cucumber and tomato	Meal 5 Vegetable Almonds	Meal 5 Fruit
			Meal 6 Walnuts	Meal 6 Vegetable		

WEST CLINIC 4 LIFE PHASE 2:
1 MONTH OF EASY EATING WEEK 2

Sunday	Monday	Tuesday	Wednesday	Thursday	Friday	Saturday
Meal 1 Oatmeal (pgs 67-68)	Meal 1 Protein Shake	Meal 1 Pancakes (pgs 70-71)	Meal 1 Breakfast Fruit Wrap (pg 73)	Meal 1 Egg whites with cooked vegetables (peppers, spinach, onions, etc.)	Meal 1 Smoothie (pg 76-78)	Meal 1 Zucchini Scrambled Eggs (pg 16)
Meal 2 Vegetable with Hummus (pg 207)	Meal 2 String cheese Fruit	Meal 2 Greek yogurt with whey protein and fruit	Meal 2 Tomato Salad (pg 56)	Meal 2 Apple with natural peanut butter	Meal 2 Cottage cheese with tomato and cucumber	Meal 2 Fruit Cottage Cheese
Meal 3 Sweet Tuna Salad (pg 133)	Meal 3 Chicken Pita Wrap (pg 134)	Meal 3 Salad (pg 90-99)	Meal 3 Salmon (pg 131-132) Steamed Vegetables	Meal 3 Vegetable with Hummus	Meal 3 Leftover pasta	Meal 3 Healthy Tortilla Chips (pg 168) with Guacamole or Pico de Gallo (pg 49)
Meal 4 Soup (pg 79-85)	Meal 4 Leftover soup	Meal 4 Chicken Fried Rice (pg 119)	Meal 4 1 Hard Boiled Egg Fruit	Meal 4 Pasta (pg 174-198)	Meal 4 Salad (pg 90-99)	Meal 4 Killer Sloppy Joes (pg 147)
Meal 5 Smoothie (pg 76-78)	Meal 5 Salad (pg 90-99)	Meal 5 Vegetable	Meal 5 Lemon Roasted Peppers (pg 59)	Meal 5 Greek yogurt with whey protein	Meal 5 String cheese	Meal 5 Great Chocolate or Vanilla Pudding (pg 224-225)
	Meal 6 Celery with natural peanut butter				Meal 6 Fruit	

WEST CLINIC 4 LIFE PHASE 2:
1 MONTH OF EASY EATING WEEK 3

Sunday	Monday	Tuesday	Wednesday	Thursday	Friday	Saturday
Meal 1 Elegant Egg White Sandwich (pg 144) Fruit	Meal 1 Pancakes (pg 70-71)	Meal 1 Banana Roll up (pg 71)	Meal 1 Greek Yogurt with whey protein powder and fruit	Meal 1 Toast with natural peanut butter Fruit	Meal 1 Simple Omelet (pg 15)	Meal 1 Oatmeal (pg 67-68)
Meal 2 Salmon (pg 131-132)	Meal 2 Avocado, tomato, and cottage cheese	Meal 2 Stuffed Zucchini (pg 211)	Meal 2 Salad (pg 90-99)	Meal 2 Kale Pomegranate Salad (pg 28)	Meal 2 Fruit Walnuts	Meal 2 Sweet and Spicy Walnut Fruit Salad (pg 90)
Meal 3 Spinach Salad (pg 27)	Meal 3 Leftover casserole	Meal 3 Chicken (pg 104-119)	Meal 3 Avocado Tuna Pita Panini (pg 136)	Meal 3 Vegetable	Meal 3 Leftover Stir Fry	Meal 3 Pizza (pg 139-157)
Meal 4 Casserole (pg 171-173)	Meal 4 Salad (pg 90-99)	Meal 4 Fruit Cottage Cheese Walnuts	Meal 4 Marinara Turkey Meatballs (pg 103)	Meal 4 Sesame Chicken Stir Fry (pg 119)	Meal 4 Spaghetti Squash Salad (pg 215)	Meal 4 Banana Bread (pg 164)
Meal 5 Zucchini Fries (pg 211)	Meal 5 Cottage Cheese with fruit	Meal 5 Healthy Tostadas (pg 160)	Meal 5 Carrots with Hummus (pg 207)	Meal 5 String Cheese	Meal 5 Greek Yogurt with whey protein	Meal 5 Salad (pg 90-99)
		Meal 6 Protein Shake				

WEST CLINIC 4 LIFE PHASE 2:
1 MONTH OF EASY EATING WEEK 4

Sunday	Monday	Tuesday	Wednesday	Thursday	Friday	Saturday
Meal 1 Leftover muffin/bread	Meal 1 So Spicy Omelet (pg 15)	Meal 1 Antioxidant Boost Yogurt (pg 73) Whole Wheat Toast	Meal 1 Oatmeal (pg 67-68)	Meal 1 Egg whites with vegetables	Meal 1 Smoothie (pg 76-78)	Meal 1 Quinoa Cinnamon Porridge (pg 75)
Meal 2 Cottage Cheese with fruit	Meal 2 Fruit String Cheese	Meal 2 2 Hard Boiled Eggs	Meal 2 String cheese Vegetable	Meal 2 Fruit	Meal 2 Salad (pg 90-99)	Meal 2 Avocado Fruit Salad (pg 32)
Meal 3 Leftover Pizza	Meal 3 (Leftover) Crispy chicken wrap with vegetables	Meal 3 Lettuce Wrap (pg 133-134)	Meal 3 Leftover Chicken Vegetable	Meal 3 Quinoa Greek Chicken Feta Salad (pg 170)	Meal 3 Cottage Cheese with tomato	Meal 3 Leftover chili
Meal 4 Salad (pg 90-99)	Meal 4 Leftover Kale Chipse	Meal 4 Fruit	Meal 4 Fruit Almonds	Meal 4 Vegetable with Hummus (pg 207)	Meal 4 Chili (pg 86-89)	Meal 4 Salad (pg 90-99)
Meal 5 Crispy Chicken Fingers (pg 108)	Meal 5 Summer Vegetable Medley (pg 212)	Meal 5 Chicken (pg 104-119) Vegetables	Meal 5 Quesadilla (pg 161)	Meal 5 Stuffed Peppers (pg 213-214)	Meal 5 Almond Broccoli Salad (pg 58)	Meal 5 Vegetable with Hummus
Meal 6 Crispy Kale Chips (pg 60)			Meal 6 Yogurt with whey protein	Meal 6 Protein Shake		

Granny's Apple Oatmeal

INGREDIENTS

2 cups old-fashioned oats

2 cups almond or rice milk

2 tablespoon of protein

½ tsp. vanilla

½ slivered almonds

½ cup no sugar added dried cranberries or other dried fruit of your choice

1 large unpeeled apple, grated

1 ½ tsp. cinnamon

4 Tbsp. 100% maple syrup, or sugar free syrup

Cooking spray

Preheat oven to 400 degrees. Coat a 3-quart (large) casserole dish or baking pan with cooking spray.

Combine all ingredients in a large bowl. If you are preparing this the night before don't add the liquid ingredients such as milk and grated apple until morning.

Place mixture in a casserole dish. Bake uncovered for 45 minutes.

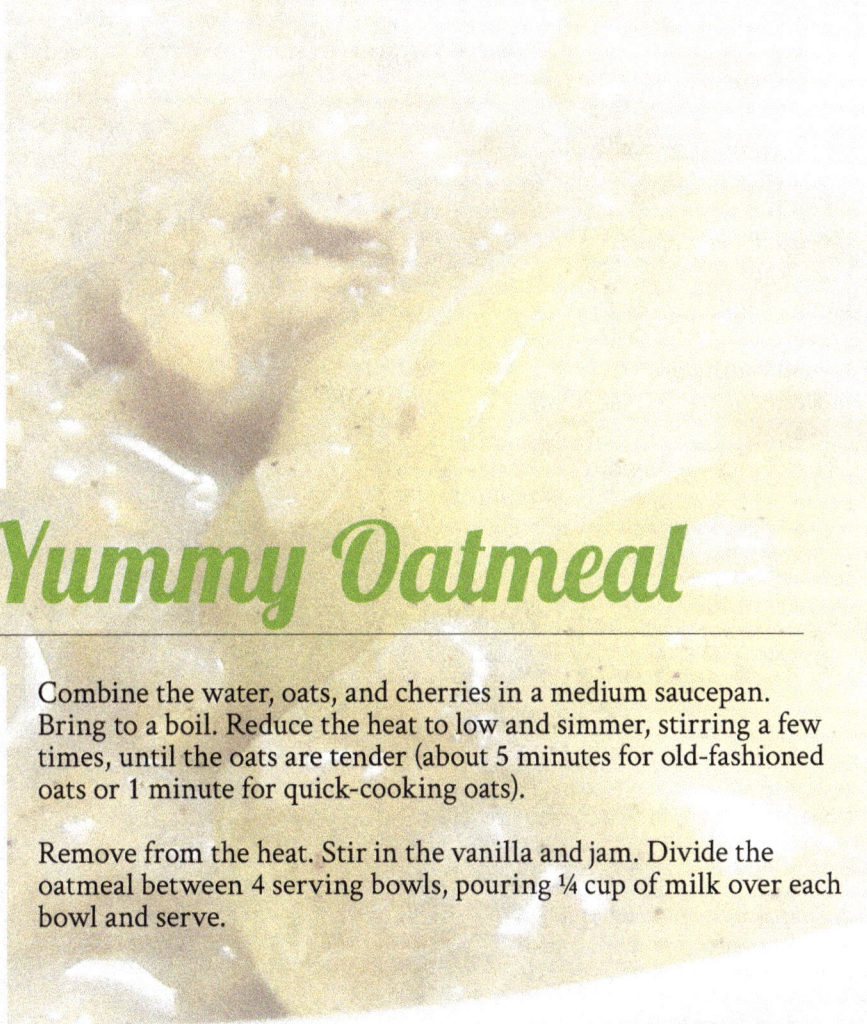

Yummy-Yummy Oatmeal

INGREDIENTS

3 ½ cups water

2 cups old-fashioned or quick-cooking rolled oats

½ cup no sugar added dried cherries

1 tsp. vanilla extract

¼ cup sugar free cherry jam (any jam flavor of your choice)

1 scoop of vanilla protein

2 Tbsp. of natural peanut, sunflower butter, or almond butter

1 cup almond or rice milk

Combine the water, oats, and cherries in a medium saucepan. Bring to a boil. Reduce the heat to low and simmer, stirring a few times, until the oats are tender (about 5 minutes for old-fashioned oats or 1 minute for quick-cooking oats).

Remove from the heat. Stir in the vanilla and jam. Divide the oatmeal between 4 serving bowls, pouring ¼ cup of milk over each bowl and serve.

Sweet Pumpkin Oatmeal

INGREDIENTS

¼ cup almond or rice milk

5 Tbsp. water

¼ cup old-fashioned oats

1 tsp. cinnamon

½ tsp. nutmeg

2 tsp. sun butter

1/8 cup canned pumpkin, unsalted

1/8 cup sliced almonds

1/8 cup water

1 scoop vanilla protein powder

1 Tbsp. Stevia (optional)

In a small pot, bring milk and water to a boil over medium heat. Add oats, sun butter, cinnamon, and nutmeg. Reduce heat to medium-low and simmer until liquid is absorbed, about 7 to 10 minutes, stirring occasionally.

Once the liquid is absorbed, stir in pumpkin, almonds, and sweetener (if desired); set aside.

Combine water and protein powder in a separate bowl. Mix with a fork until protein is dissolved. For a smoother consistency, mix powder with water in a blender or food processor and blend until protein is dissolved. If sweetener is desired, choose Stevia.

Pour protein mixture over oatmeal and serve.

Creamy Oatmeal

INGREDIENTS

2/3 cup quick-cooking oats

2 Tbsp. raisins

1 1/3 cup apple juice

1 ½ tsp. cinnamon

½ tsp. vanilla extract

¼ cup Greek yogurt

1, 4-cup microwavable measuring cup, stir oats, raisins, apple juice, cinnamon, and vanilla extract until well blended.

Microwave on High 2-3 minutes, stirring every 30 seconds, until thickened. Top each serving with yogurt.

Sunshine Pumpkin Muffins

INGREDIENTS

1 cup old-fashioned oatmeal, not instant

½ cup unsweetened applesauce

½ cup canned pumpkin*

2 large egg whites + 1 yolk, lightly beaten

2 Tbsp. + 1 tsp. olive oil

1 Tbsp. double-acting baking powder

½ tsp. baking soda

2 tsp. cinnamon

½ tsp. ground nutmeg

1 ½ tsp. pumpkin pie spice

½ cup almond or rice milk or ½ cup apple juice

½ cup amaranth or quinoa flour

¼ cup whole-wheat flour

¼ cup no sugar added dried cranberries or raisins (optional)

*If you don't have pumpkin you can use a sweet potato. Simply microwave the sweet potato and let cool. Remove the skin and mash the flesh. Measure out the required quantity.

Method:

Preheat oven to 375 degrees. Line muffin pan with paper or silicon liners or coat with cooking spray.

Combine oatmeal, pumpkin, applesauce, juice or milk, eggs, and oil. Mix until all ingredients are blended.

Measure and mix all dry ingredients. Make a well in the center and pour wet ingredients into dry.

Add dried fruit if using. Mix until dry ingredients are just moistened. Fill muffin cups 2/3 full. Bake 15-20 minutes or until lightly browned on top.

Fun Fact: We, as a society, are addicted to sugar. On average, we consume about 22.2 teaspoons (roughly a half a cup) of sugar every day - 182.5 cups every year.

Gluten-Free Pancake Treats

INGREDIENTS

1 cup flour

1/4 cup tapioca

1 ½ tsp. guar gum

3/4 cup rice flour

½ cup almond or rice milk

1 tsp. organic honey or Stevia

1 tsp. cinnamon

2 eggs or egg white substitute

1 Tbsp. canola, coconut or safflower oil

Place all dry ingredients in a medium bowl.

Using a whisk, mix dry ingredients well. Add milk, honey/Stevia, eggs, and oil. Whisk until all ingredients are well blended. Add more milk if necessary to make batter runny.

Pour ¼ to 1/3 cup pancake batter on hot griddle or frying pan coated with cooking spray. When bubbles form on top of pancake, flip. Cook until golden on both sides.

Protein-Loaded Pancakes

INGREDIENTS

2 large ripe bananas

2 Tbsp. cinnamon

2 tsp. vanilla extract

1 cup old fashion oats

2 scoops vanilla protein powder

2 (8 oz.) cartons of egg substitute or 14 egg whites

Sugar Free Syrup

In a blender, add all of the ingredients (except the syrup) in order. Blend for 8-10 seconds.

In a blender add all of the ingredients. In a non-stick frying pan, over medium heat, pour 4-inch by 4- inch pancakes. Flip when you see air bubbles on the top. Cook on the second side uncovered until the bottom is golden brown.

Berry Pancakes

INGREDIENTS

½ cup almond or rice milk

½ cup whole grain oat flour

1 large egg white, lightly beaten

½ tsp. baking soda

¼ tsp. vanilla extract

½ cup fresh or frozen berries of your choice

In a small bowl, combine milk, flour, egg whites, baking soda, and vanilla. Whisk until blended. Stir in the blueberries or berries of your choice. Let stand for 10 minutes.

Heat a large non-stick skillet over medium heat. Pour batter in 1/8 cup dollops onto skillet to form 4 pancakes. Cook 2 minutes until bubbles form on top and the bottom is golden brown. Flip and cook 2 more minutes or until bottom is golden brown.

Banana Roll-ups

INGREDIENTS

8 oz. package fat-free cream cheese, softened

2 Tbsp. agave nectar or raw honey

1 Tbsp. cinnamon

1 tsp. nutmeg, ground

Olive oil cooking spray

2 large ripe bananas, sliced

4-100% whole wheat tortillas

Topping Ingredients (Optional):

1 banana, sliced

¼ cup fresh mint

¼ cup agave nectar

In a medium mixing bowl, combine cream cheese, agave nectar or honey, cinnamon, and nutmeg, stirring well.

Heat a large nonstick skillet coated with cooking spray over medium-high heat. Spread 1 Tbsp. cream cheese mixture and place half of each banana on top of each tortilla; roll up tortillas. Place 2 roll-ups in skillet and cook 2 minutes per side or until tortillas are lightly browned and crisp. Remove from pan and keep warm. Repeat procedure with remaining roll-ups. Cut each roll-up in half.

If desired, prepare topping: Heat additional banana slices in large nonstick skillet for 1 to 2 minutes per side or until lightly browned. Top roll-ups with additional banana slices, mint, and agave nectar.

SERVES

8

Lean Morning Bars

INGREDIENTS

2 cups puffed wheat

1/3 cup ground almonds or walnuts

2 Tbsp. ground flaxseeds

1 cup vanilla whey protein powder

1/3 cup dried unsweetened fruit (cranberries, blueberries, or raisins)

1/3 cup pure maple syrup or agave nectar

1 Tbsp. coconut oil

1 tsp. vanilla extract

2 Tbsp. natural peanut butter

Olive oil cooking spray

In a bowl, combine dry ingredients. Set aside.

In a pot, combine syrup or agave nectar and coconut oil. Heat to a simmer. Add vanilla extract and peanut butter and remove from heat. Stir with a fork to blend ingredients.

Add liquid mixture to cereal mixture and mix with a spoon.

Press evenly into an oiled 8-by-8-inch pan. Let cool in the refrigerator until solid. Cut into 8 squares.

Wrap individually and keep frozen for best results.

SERVES
8

Oatmeal Protein Breakfast Bars

INGREDIENTS

2 ¼ cups old-fashioned oats

½ cup honey or Stevia

¾ cup of raisins or any other fruit (apples, bananas, blueberries, etc.)/nuts

1 ½ Tbsp. cinnamon

3 1/3 cup almond or rice milk

4 egg whites lightly beaten

½ cup vanilla protein

1 tsp. olive oil

1 tsp. vanilla extract

Heat oven to 350 degrees.

Combine the dry ingredients into the wet and mix. Pour into sprayed 8 inch baking dish and bake for about 40-45 minutes, making sure it does not dry out.

Breakfast Fruit Wraps

INGREDIENTS

½ cup Natural Peanut Butter or Sunflower Butter

4 whole wheat tortillas (8 to 10 inch)

¼ cup honey or Stevia

2 small bananas, sliced

1 ½ tsp. cinnamon

Spread 2 Tbsp. of peanut butter or sunflower butter spread evenly over each tortilla. Drizzle 1 Tbsp. honey/Stevia over each tortilla. Top with banana slices. Roll up tortillas and secure with toothpicks.

Antioxidant Boost Yogurt

INGREDIENTS

1 cup fat-free quark, kefir, or Greek yogurt

½ cup almond or rice milk

1 tsp. lemon juice

1 Tbsp. organic honey

2 Tbsp. flax oil

1 ½ Tbsp. ground flax seeds

1 unpeeled, grated apple

1 Tbsp. coarsely grated walnuts

1 ½ tsp. cinnamon

½ cup blueberries, divided

½ cup raspberries, divided

In a medium bowl blend the quark/kefir/Greek yogurt with almond/ rice milk, lemon juice, honey, flax oil, and cinnamon. Set aside.

Spoon 1 Tbsp. of ground flax seed in each of two smaller cereal bowls. Do the same with the apples, ground walnuts and berries. Divide mixture in first bowl evenly between the two smaller bowls.

Muesli Mix

INGREDIENTS

½ cup hot water

½ cup 3-5 minutes oats

1 cup fat-free Greek yogurt

¼ cup raisins

¼ cup no sugar added dried cherries or cranberries

2 Tbsp. natural bran

2 Tbsp. wheat germ

2 Tbsp. coarsely ground flax seeds

2 Tbsp. oat bran

2 Tbsp. Stevia

1 tsp. cinnamon

1 apple, unpeeled, cored and diced

3 bananas, peeled and sliced

In a medium bowl, pour hot water over oats. Let stand for 20 minutes or until water is absorbed.

Add remaining ingredients except bananas. Mix well. Cover and refrigerate for up to three days.

Serve with sliced bananas.

SERVES

4

Quinoa Cinnamon Porridge

INGREDIENTS

½ cup uncooked quinoa

1 cup water

1 ½ tsp. cinnamon

½ cup almond or rice milk

1 apple, diced

½ cup blueberries or sliced strawberries

1/8 cup chopped pecans or walnuts

Agave syrup (optional)

1 tsp. vanilla extract

Add quinoa, water, and cinnamon to a small pot and bring to a boil. Reduce heat, cover, and simmer for 15 minutes or until most of water has been absorbed. Add milk and simmer uncovered for an additional 10 minutes. Stir in apple, berries, nuts, and vanilla. Cover and let sit for 10 minutes before serving. Porridge will thicken during this time. If desired, drizzle with agave syrup before serving.

SERVES

2

Christine's Frittata

INGREDIENTS

1½ -2 Tbsp. extra-virgin olive oil

1 clove garlic, minced

½ onion, chopped

2 cups fresh spinach, chopped

1/3 cup sundried tomatoes, chopped

4 organic eggs + 4 egg whites, beaten

2 oz. fat-free mozzarella cheese

2 Tbsp. shredded parmesan

Add any lean meat of choice

Preheat oven to 400 degrees. Heat olive oil over medium-high heat. Add onions and garlic until tender. Add spinach and sundried tomatoes 1 to 2 minutes until spinach is wilted.

Reduce heat and add eggs and cheese, season to taste. Cover and cook over medium heat 5-7 minutes until eggs set up. Uncover and place in preheated oven 5 minutes until top is firm.

SERVES

4

Breakfast On-the-Go

INGREDIENTS

1 scoop protein powder, vanilla or chocolate

1/3 cup dry oatmeal

2/3 cup water or, almond or rice milk

1 Tbsp. natural almond butter or natural peanut butter or sunflower butter

1 frozen banana (can use fresh if no frozen are available)

2 Tbsp. unsweetened applesauce

1 ½ tsp. cinnamon

1 Tbsp. ground flax seed

1 ½ Tbsp. wheat germ

¾ cup ice cubes

Blend all ingredients.

Protein-Packed Smoothie

Puree all ingredients, adding ice to adjust consistency of smoothie.

INGREDIENTS

¼ cup dry, uncooked oatmeal

1 Tbsp. natural peanut butter or sunflower butter

1 scoop protein powder

1 ½ Tbsp. organic honey or agave nectar

1 Tbsp. flax seed

1 cup almond or rice milk

1 tsp. cinnamon

Handful of ice cubes

Crazy Kiwi Smoothie

INGREDIENTS

1 kiwi, peeled

1 navel orange, peeled

1 scoop whey protein powder

½ cup fat-free Greek yogurt

1 tsp. lemon flavored avocado oil

½ tsp. nutmeg

1 tsp. cinnamon

1 tsp. fresh lime juice

½ cup ice cubes

Puree all ingredients. If the smoothie is too thick add more ice and blend again.

Easy Smoothie

INGREDIENTS

½ cup fat-free Greek yogurt

½ cup almond or rice milk

1 tsp. vanilla extract

1 ½ tsp. lemon-flavored avocado oil

1 ½ scoops whey protein (any flavor)

1 orange, peeled

1 Tbsp. wheat germ

½ banana

Handful of ice cubes

Puree all ingredients.

Blue Razz Smoothie

INGREDIENTS

½ cup almond or rice milk

1/3 cup water

½ cup frozen blueberries

1 Tbsp. flax seed

½ cup unsweetened applesauce

½ cup fat-free Greek yogurt

1-2 scoops whey protein powder (any flavor)

Handful of ice cubes

Puree all ingredients.

Berry Spinach Smoothie

INGREDIENTS

1 heaping cup of spinach

½ cup raspberries

½ cup blueberries

4-5 strawberries

1 scoop whey protein powder

1 cup cold water

2 Tbsp. Greek yogurt

Handful of ice cubes

Puree all ingredients.

Garlicky Tomato Soup

INGREDIENTS

3 medium garlic cloves, peeled and minced

3 Tbsp. of olive oil

2 lbs Italian plum tomatoes, peeled, seeded, and chopped

1 ¼ quarts chicken broth

5 basil leaves, chopped

In a large pot, sauté garlic in olive oil over low heat

Add tomatoes and cook on low heat, uncovered for 10 minutes stirring frequently

Add chicken broth and let simmer for 20 minutes

Stir in basil

SERVES
4

Great Green Soup

INGREDIENTS

2 head broccoli, stem ends trimmed

3 Tbsp. unsalted butter

1 large onion, diced

2 leeks, sliced thin

4 cloves of garlic, minced

6 cups chicken stock

2 ripe plum tomatoes, chopped

1 bunch fresh spinach leaves

¼ cup chopped parsley

¼ cup fresh lemon juice

Chop broccoli florets and slice stem thin

Melt butter in soup kettle, add onions and garlic, cook on low for 10 minutes

Add the chicken stock, broccoli, tomatoes, and parsley. Bring to a boil, reduce heat, and then cover for 25 minutes to simmer.

Add spinach to soup and cook for 1 minute longer, then remove from heat and allow to slightly cool.

Puree soup in batches in blender or food processor. Return pureed soup to pot and heat. Add lemon juice just before serving.

SERVES
8

Spicy Black Bean Soup

INGREDIENTS

2 Tbsp. extra virgin olive oil

2 ribs celery, trimmed and coarsely chopped

1 large carrot, peeled and chopped

1 small red onion, peeled and chopped

1 red pepper, seeded, de-veined, and chopped

1 green pepper, seeded, de-veined, and chopped

2 garlic cloves, finely chopped

1 Tbsp. dried cumin

1 ½ tsp. dried oregano

2 tsp. dried basil

1 Tbsp. chili powder

2 Tbsp. Frank's hot sauce

4 cups low-sodium chicken or vegetable stock (gluten free if necessary)

2-15oz. cans black beans

1-15oz. canned no salt added diced tomatoes or fresh Roma tomatoes

1 cup fresh corn kernels

In a large skillet, heat olive oil over medium heat. Add celery, carrot, onion, and bell peppers. Sauté until onion becomes translucent, about 8 minutes. Add garlic and spices. Cook another 2 minutes.

Add stock or cooking liquid of your choice, beans, tomatoes, and corn. Bring mixture to a boil and then reduce heat. Cover and let simmer for about 20 minutes. Using a hand-held blender, puree soup to desired consistency. Add corn and let simmer for 5 minutes. Season with Mrs. Dash spices. Serve hot.

SERVES

8

Research has shown that most, if not all chronic disease is directly caused from inflammation in the body. Inflammation has been directly connected to sugar. Logic tells us that if inflammation is the cause of chronic disease, and if we decrease the amount of sugar in our diets, then we have a very good chance of decreasing chronic disease.

French Onion Soup

INGREDIENTS

2 Tbsp. extra-virgin olive oil

2 cups red onion, finely diced and sliced

1 ½ cups sweet, yellow onion, finely diced and sliced

½ cup white onion, finely diced and sliced

2 Tbsp. unfiltered, fresh apple cider

1 ½ Tbsp. whole-wheat flour

8 cups certified organic low-sodium chicken broth

Heat a large pot over medium-high heat for 1 minute. Add oil and heat for another minute. Reduce

heat to medium-low and add onions, sauté, stirring occasionally with lid half-covering pot, about 20 minutes. Onions will slowly caramelize.

Add apple cider and stir to deglaze. Add flour and stir to thicken. Then add broth. Increase heat to medium-high; simmer 10 minutes. Reduce heat to low or turn off until ready to serve.

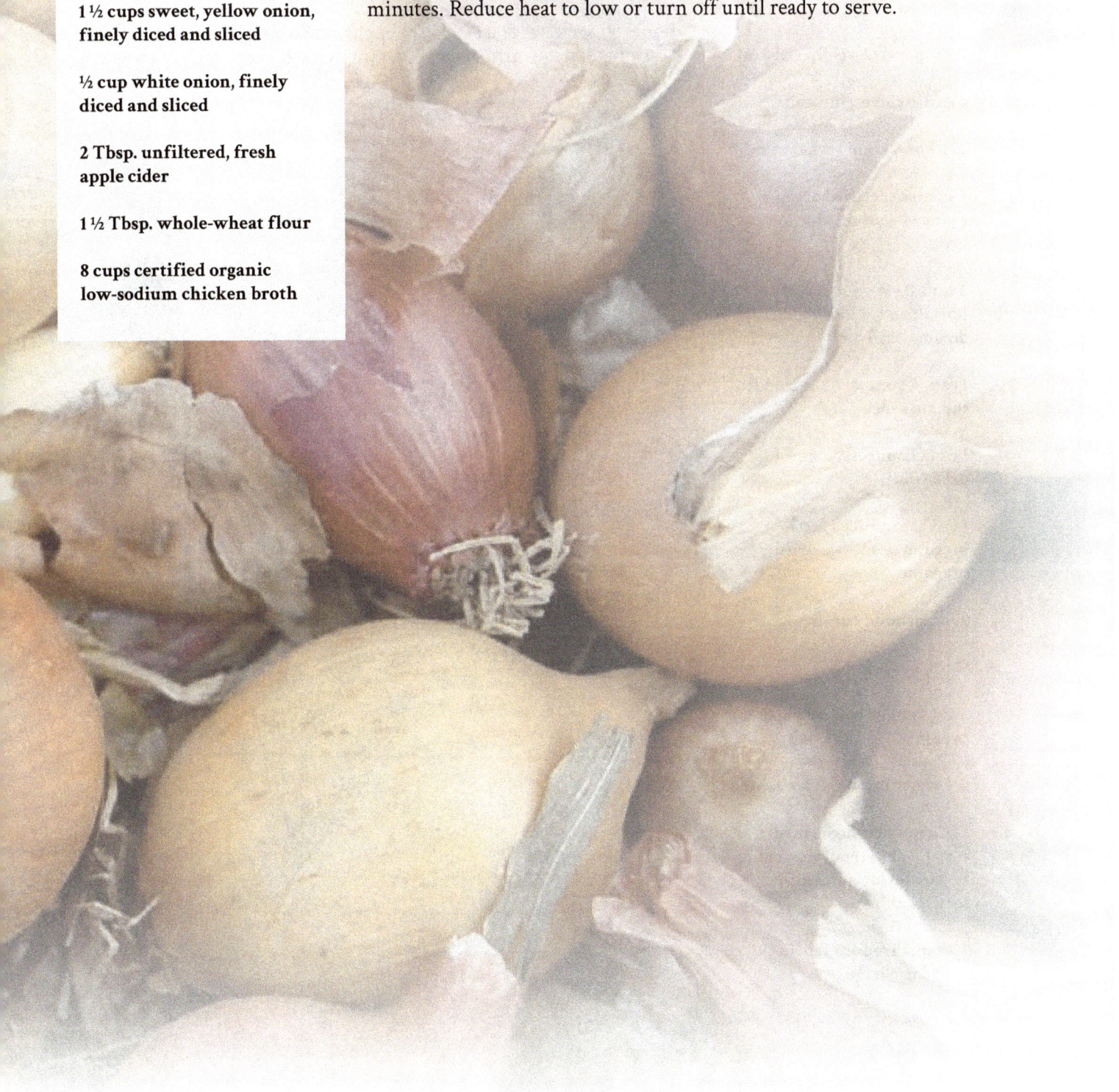

Tortilla Mexican Soup

INGREDIENTS

1 large onion, chopped

2 green onions, thinly chopped

2 Tbsp. extra-virgin olive oil

4 garlic cloves, minced

2 ½ Tbsp. whole-wheat flour

4 ½ cups certified organic reduced-sodium chicken broth

2 cans (14 ½ ounces each) no-salt added diced tomatoes, do not drain

1 can (8 ounces) no-salt added tomato sauce

1 can (4 ounces) chopped green chilies

1 ½ Tbsp. minced fresh oregano or 1 ½ tsp. dried oregano

2 tsp. ground cumin

¼ tsp. pepper

3 cups cubed cooked chicken breast

4 Tbsp. minced fresh cilantro

1 1/3 cups crushed baked tortilla chip scoops (refer to page 60 for homemade tortilla chips)

7 Tbsp. shredded fat-free cheddar cheese

In a Dutch oven, sauté onion and green onions in olive oil until tender. Add garlic; sauté 2 minutes longer.

Stir in flour until blended; gradually add broth. Stir in the tomatoes, tomato sauce, chilies, oregano, cumin, and pepper. Bring to a boil. Reduce heat; cover and simmer for 20 minutes. Add chicken and cilantro; heat through.

For each serving, place 2 Tbsp. of chips in a soup bowl. Top with 1 ½ cups soup. Garnish each serving with 1 Tbsp. each of cheese and chips.

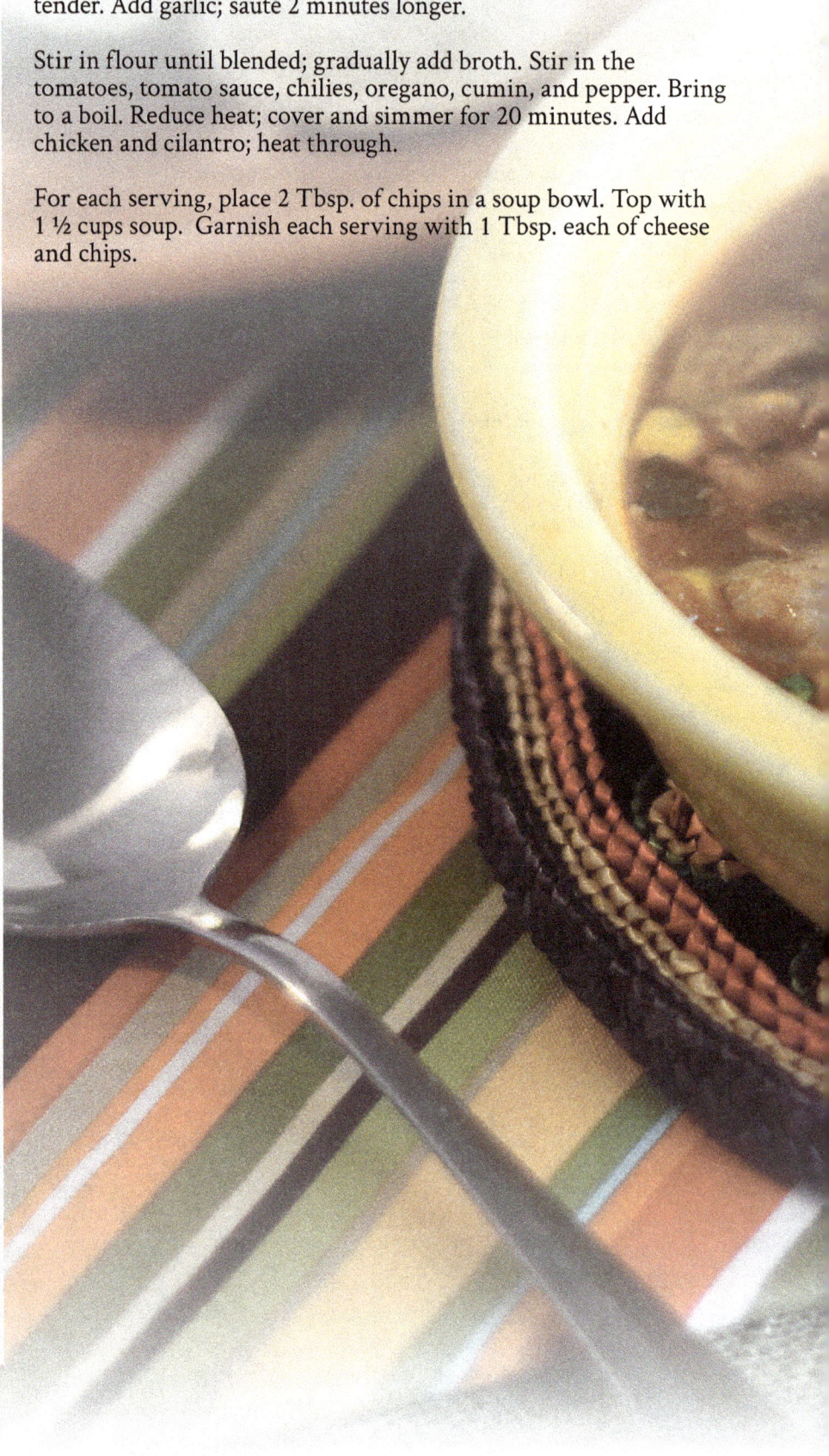

Creamy Pumpkin Soup

INGREDIENTS

2 tsp. olive oil

1 clove garlic, minced

1 inch ginger, peeled and minced

2 medium Vidalia onions, diced

2 tsp. curry powder

2 cups "certified organic" reduced-sodium vegetable stock

¼ cup reduced-fat coconut milk

1 can (15 ounces) unsalted pumpkin, puree

1/3 cup calcium-fortified orange juice

1/8 tsp. ground nutmeg

1/8 tsp. cayenne pepper

Toasted pumpkin seeds (optional)

In a heavy saucepan, heat oil over medium-low heat. Stir in garlic, onions, ginger, curry powder, and cook for 1 minute, until fragrant.

Add vegetable stock and coconut milk and turn heat to medium. Stir in pumpkin puree and orange juice until well blended.

Stir soup occasionally until heated through, about 5 minutes. Take soup off the heat and stir in nutmeg, and cayenne pepper. Garnish bowls of soup with toasted pumpkin seeds, if desired.

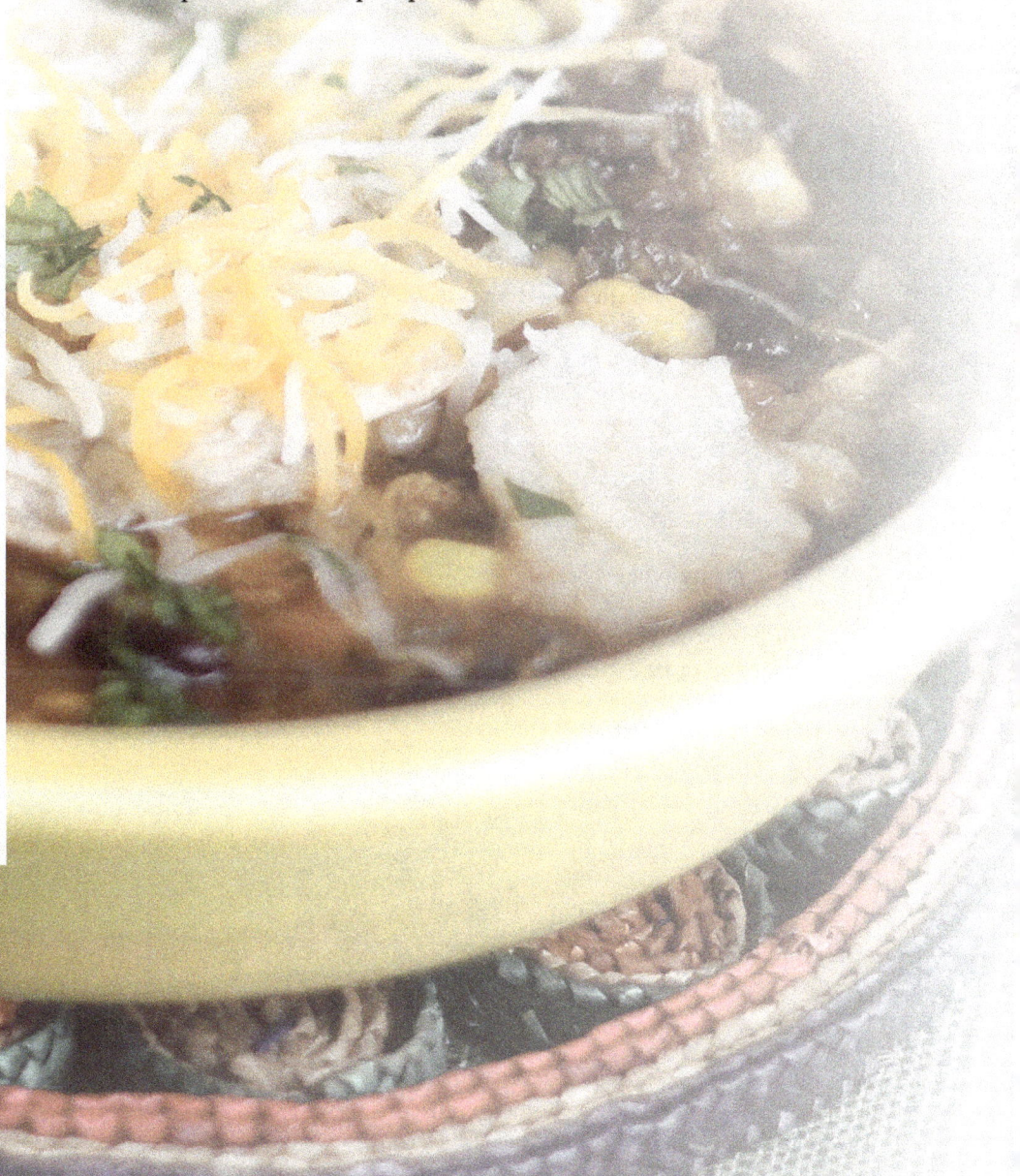

Easy Bee Soup

INGREDIENTS

½ pound lean ground beef

2 large fresh mushrooms, sliced

1 celery rib, chopped

1 small onion, chopped

2 tsp. whole-wheat flour

3 cans (14 ½ ounces each) reduced-sodium beef broth

2 medium carrots, sliced

1 large potato, peeled and cubed

1/8 tsp. salt

1 tsp. pepper

1/3 cup medium pearl barley

1 can (5 ounces) fat-free evaporated milk

3 Tbsp. tomato paste

In a Dutch oven over medium heat, cook and stir the beef, mushrooms, celery, and onion until meat is no longer pink; drain. Stir in flour until blended; gradually add broth. Stir in the carrots, potato, pepper, and salt. Bring to a boil. Stir in barley.

Reduce heat; cover and simmer for 45-50 minutes or until barley is tender. Whisk in milk and tomato paste; heat through.

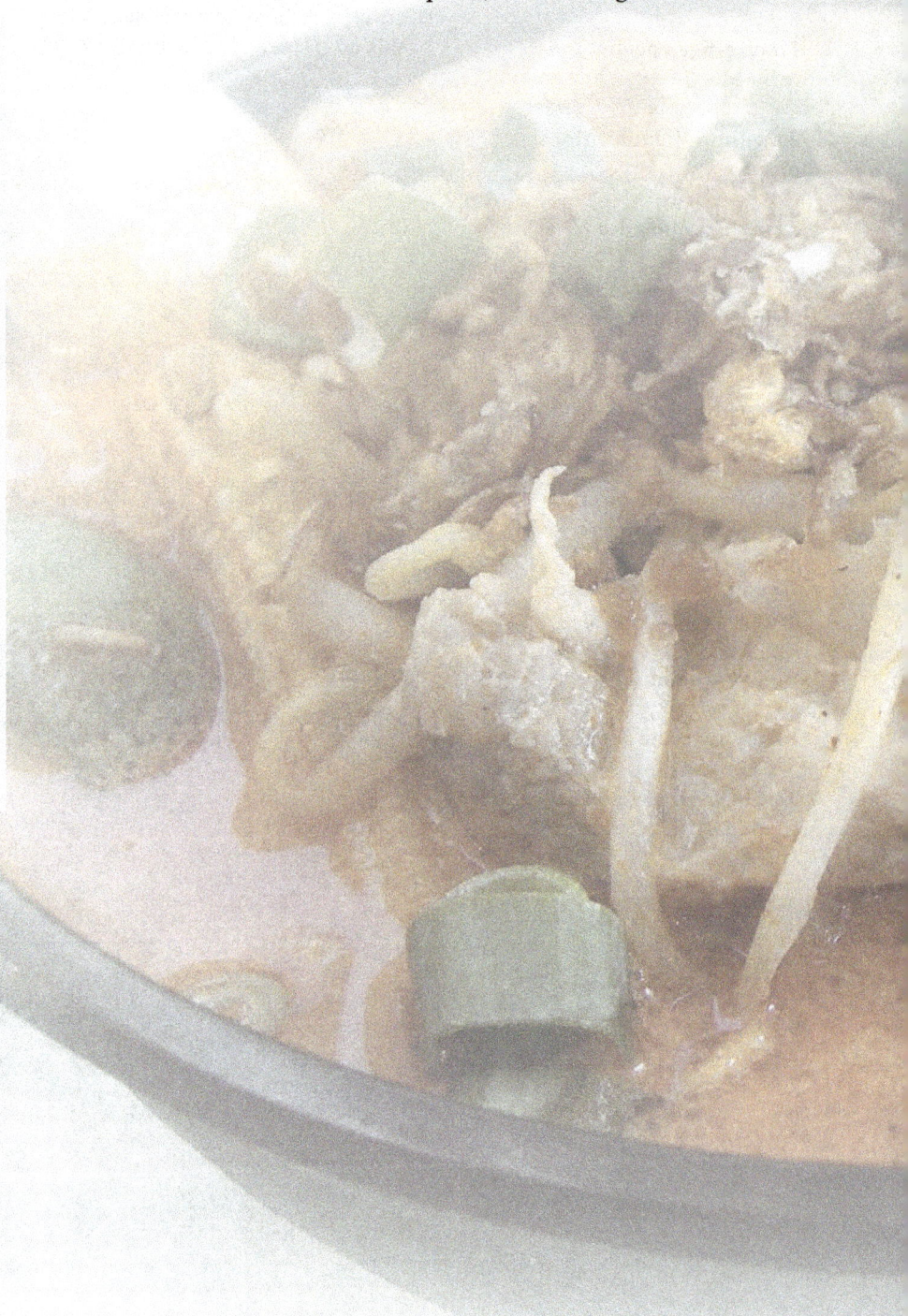

Curry Soup

INGREDIENTS

2 ounces whole wheat or gluten-free linguini noodles

1 Tbsp. extra virgin olive oil

1 clove garlic, minced

1 ½ Tbsp. lemon grass, minced

2 tsp. ground ginger

2 tsp. red curry paste

1 (32 ounce) carton reduced-sodium chicken broth

2 Tbsp. low-sodium soy sauce

1 (13 ½ ounce) can reduced-fat coconut milk

½ cup peeled and deveined medium shrimp or 2 boneless, skinless chicken breasts

½ cup sliced mushrooms

1 (10 ounce) bag baby spinach leaves

2 Tbsp. fresh lime juice

½ cup chopped cilantro

3 green onions, thinly sliced

Bring a large pot of lightly salted water to a boil. Add rice noodles and cook until tender, about 3 minutes. Drain and rinse well with cold water to stop the cooking; set aside.

Heat oil in a large saucepan over medium heat. Stir in garlic, lemon grass, and ginger; cook and stir until aromatic, 30-60 seconds. Add the curry paste, and cook 30 seconds more. Pour in about ½ cup of the chicken broth, and stir until the curry paste has dissolved, then pour in the remaining chicken stock along with the soy sauce. Bring to a boil, then reduce heat to medium-low, partially cover, and simmer 20 minutes.

Stir in coconut milk, shrimp/chicken, mushrooms, spinach, lime juice, and cilantro. Increase heat to medium-high, and simmer until the shrimp turn pink and are no longer translucent, about 5 minutes/chicken turn golden brown.

To serve, place some linguini noodles into each serving bowl and ladle soup on top of them. Garnish each bowl with a sprinkle of sliced green onion.

SERVES

4

Loaded Chili

INGREDIENTS

1 box of whole wheat spaghetti

1 container of fat-free Greek Yogurt (use as sour cream topping)

1 Tbsp. fat-free mozzarella cheese or 2 Tbsp. reduced-fat parmesan cheese

2 cans of light red kidney beans

1 lb of 93% or better, lean ground beef, or ground turkey burger

4 ½ Tbsp. no salt chili powder

2 Tbsp. cayenne pepper

1 red onion

6 small cans of no salt added tomato sauce

1 small can of no salt added tomato paste

1 can of water from bean can

1 ½ Tbsp. minced garlic

2 Tbsp. oregano

1 Tbsp. Italian seasoning

½ tsp. extra-virgin olive oil

Cook meat and set aside. Cook pasta rinse in cold water and set aside. Chop onion and add half to sauce, and set other half aside. Add tomato sauce, paste, water, powder, seasoning, beans, garlic, and start to heat on medium heat. Stir often to avoid burning. Once there is a light boil add meat and simmer for 20 minutes. Remove from heat. Add ½ tsp. of oil to noodles and heat for 20 seconds in microwave. Add chili over a serving of noodles, and top with cheese, onion, and Greek yogurt.

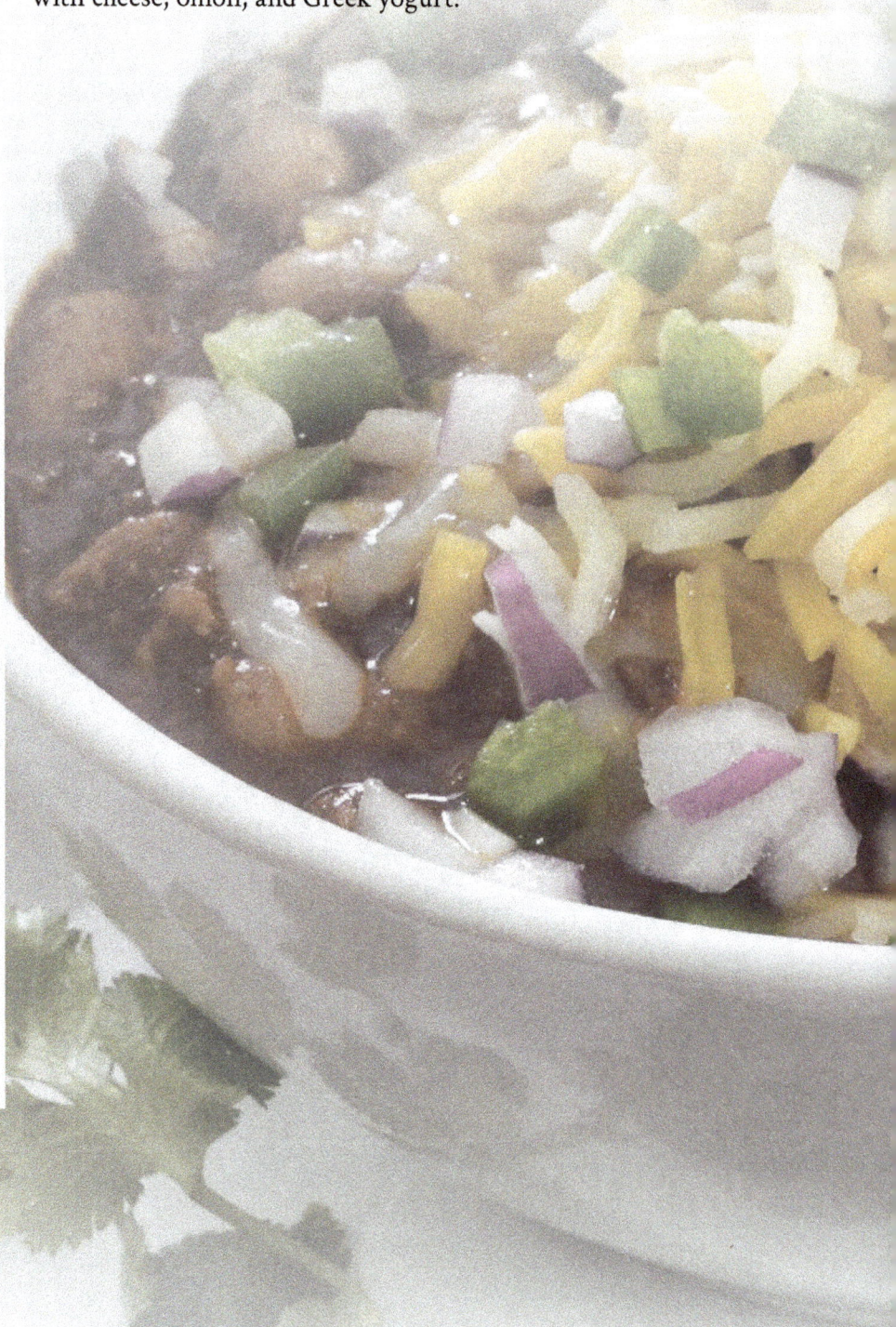

Christmas Chili

INGREDIENTS

1 lb. boneless, skinless chicken breasts

1 can Cannellini or Great Northern beans

1 can light red kidney beans

4 cup spinach

2 Tbsp. chili powder

Mrs. Dash spices and garlic, onions, and basil to taste

Cook chicken and season to taste, add powder and one cup of water, beans, and bring to a boil.

Then reduce heat to a simmer and add spinach. Cook for two more minutes while stirring lightly.

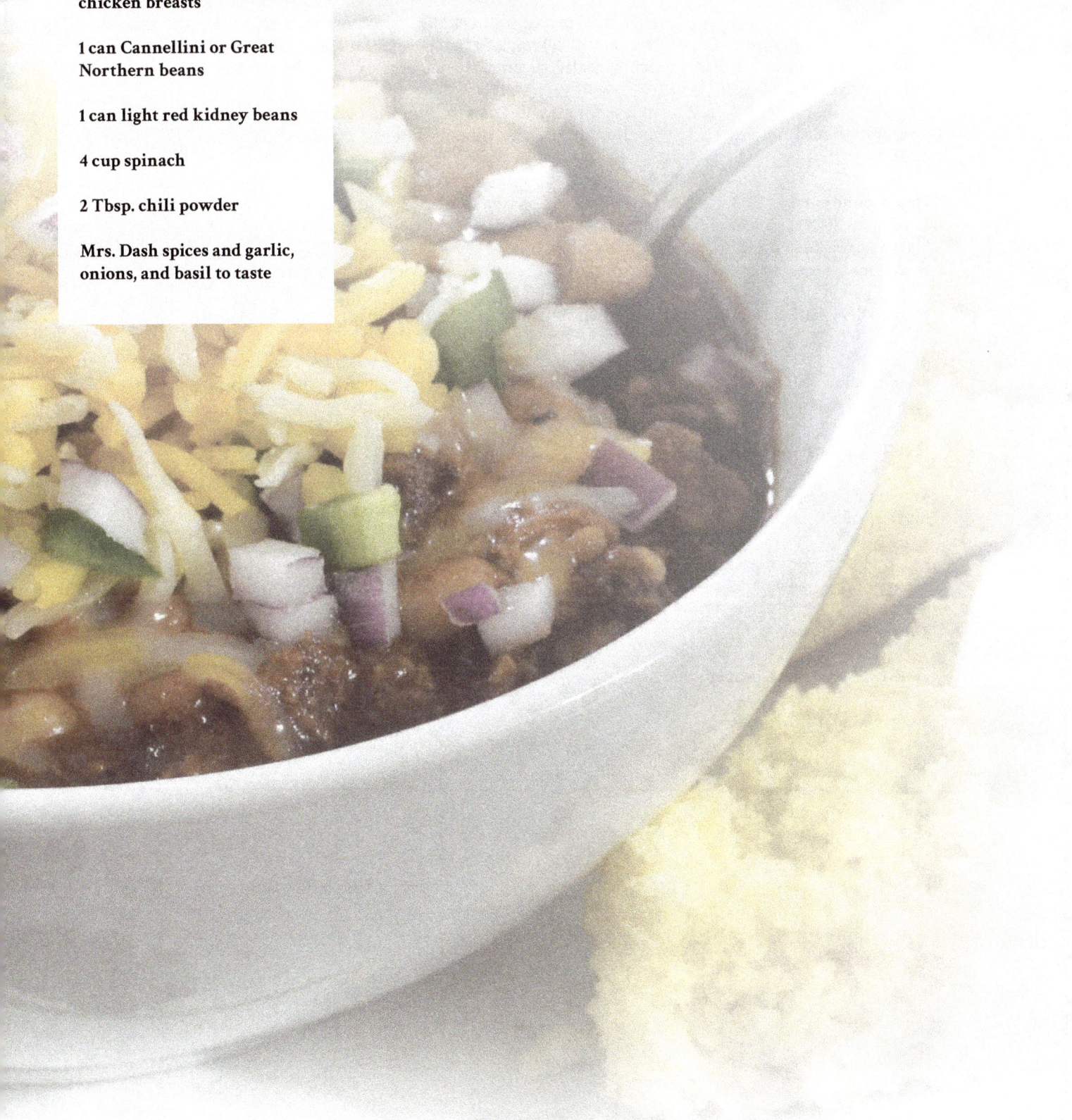

Vegetable with Ground Turkey Chili

INGREDIENTS

1 ½ Tbsp. extra virgin olive oil

1 large onion, medium diced

2 garlic clove, minced

1 red chili, seeded and small diced

1 tsp. ground cumin

1 large carrot, peeled and small diced

1 large celery stalk, medium diced

1 small yellow bell pepper, seeded and medium diced

12 oz. 1% lean ground turkey

4 medium size ripe tomatoes, medium diced

8 oz. cooked white or black beans

4 cups baby spinach

Freshly ground black pepper

¼ cup plain fat-free Greek yogurt

Cilantro to garnish (can substitute with chopped chives)

Place a large sauté pan over medium high heat, then drizzle with the oil.

Add the onion, garlic, and red chili and sauté for 2 minutes, or until tender.

Sprinkle the cumin over the onion mix and stir well, then add the carrot, celery, and bell pepper and cook for 5 minutes, stirring occasionally, or until the vegetables begin to get tender.

In a separate sauté pan, brown the turkey in the remaining oil over medium high heat, then transfer to the vegetable mix.

Add the tomatoes and the beans and cook for a further 8 minutes, stirring occasionally, or until the tomatoes have broken down and most of the liquid has evaporated.

Stir in the spinach and remove from the heat.

Season the chili to taste with freshly ground black pepper.

Spoon the chili onto serving dishes and spoon a Tbsp. of the yogurt onto each garnish with the cilantro (or chives) and serve.

SERVES

4

Protein Loaded Chili

INGREDIENTS

1 lb. lean ground beef

1 medium onion, chopped

1 medium green pepper, chopped

1 ¾ cups water

2 cans (8 ounces each) no salt added tomato sauce

1 can (16 ounces) kidney beans, rinsed and drained

1 can (15.5 ounces) great northern beans, rinsed and drained

1 can (15 ounces) garbanzo beans or chickpeas, rinsed and drained

1 can (15 ounces) black beans, rinsed and drained

1 Tbsp. baking cocoa

2 ½ tsp. Louisiana-style hot sauce

½ tsp. pepper

1 tsp. chili powder

½ tsp. garlic powder

½ tsp. cayenne pepper

½ cup fat-free Greek yogurt

½ cup crushed homemade tortilla chip (sliced up tortilla strips and baked in oven for 10 minutes.)

½ cup shredded fat-free cheddar cheese

In a Dutch oven over medium heat, cook the beef, onion, and pepper until meat is no longer pink; drain.

Stir in the water, tomato sauce, beans, cocoa, hot sauce, and seasonings. Bring to a boil. Reduce heat; cover and simmer for 30 minutes. Garnish each serving with 1 Tbsp. each of Greek yogurt, crushed homemade tortilla chips, and cheeses.

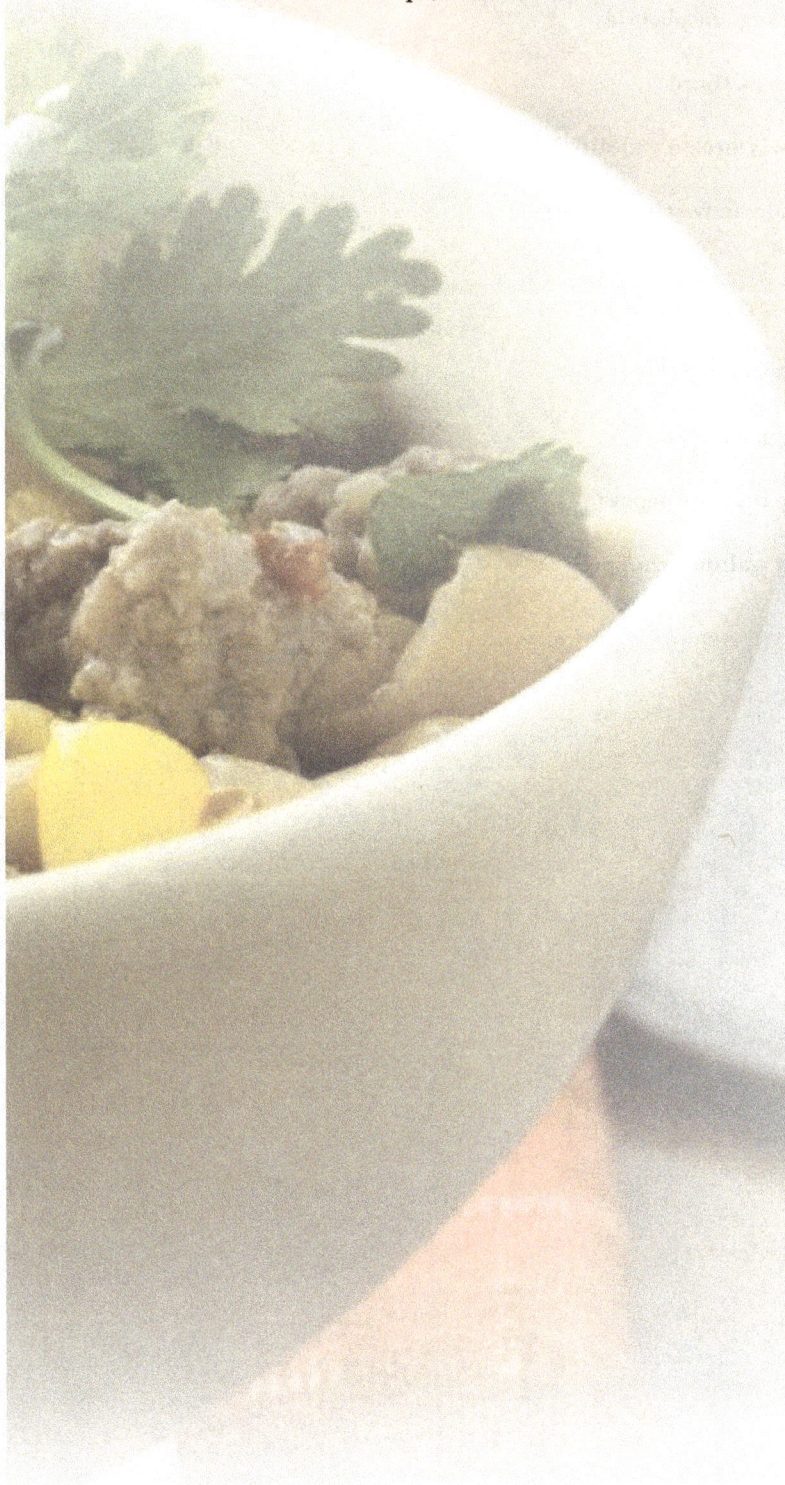

Sweet and Spicy Walnut Fruit Salad

INGREDIENTS

1 package strawberries, halved

1 package raspberries

1 mango, sliced

3 kiwis, peeled and sliced

2 apples (any color/brand), wedges

1 nectarine, chopped

1 Tbsp. honey

1 Tbsp. hot water

¾ tsp cayenne pepper

1 cup walnuts, chopped

In a large bowl, combine all fruit.

In a small bowl, combine honey, hot water, and cayenne. Mix well. Add walnuts and stir until well coated. Place walnuts on baking sheet and broil for 1-3 minutes (watch them so they do not burn).

Stir walnuts into fruit before serving.

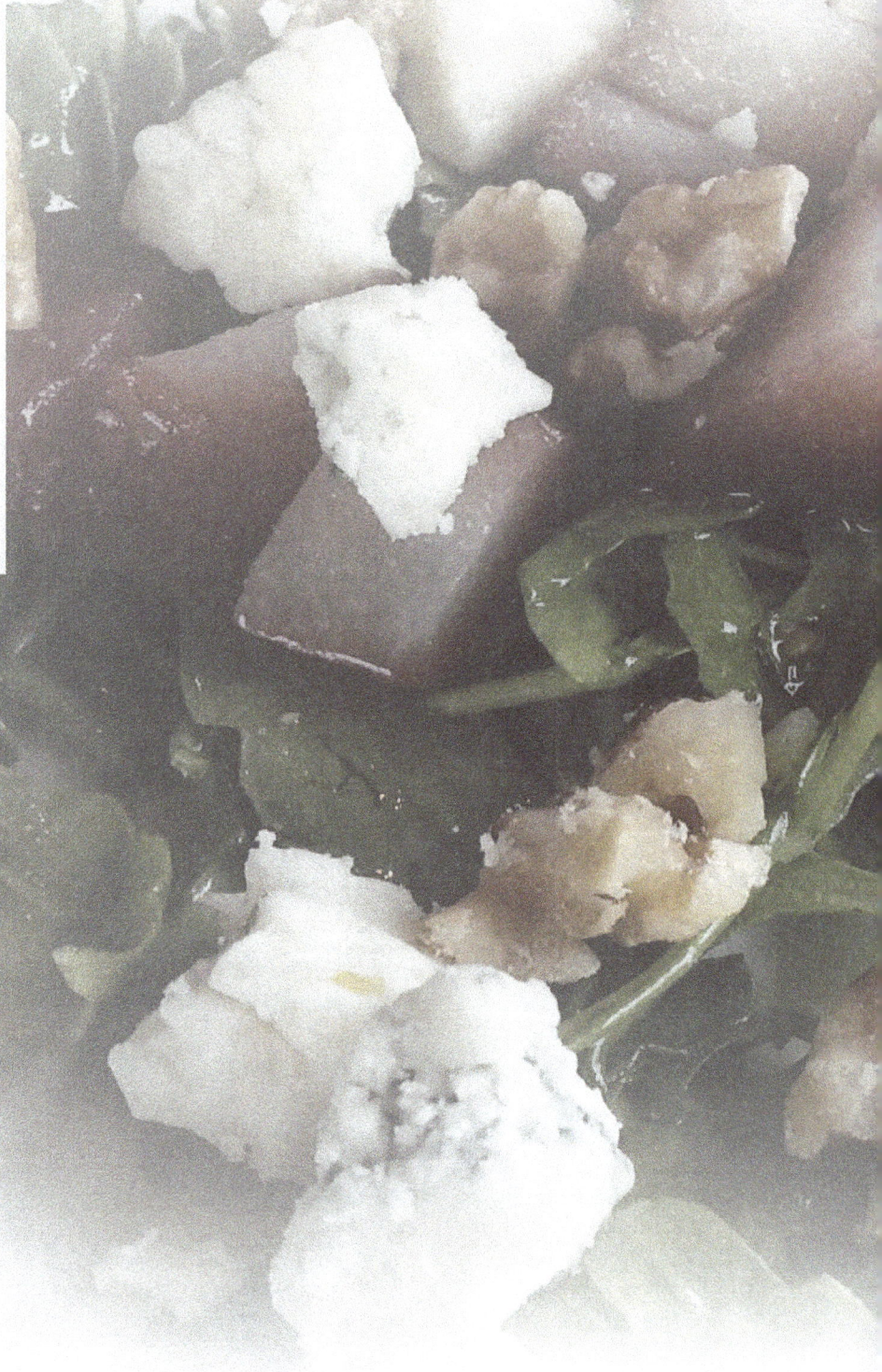

Ginger-Soy Vinaigrette Salad

INGREDIENTS

Vinaigrette Ingredients:

1 Tbsp. fresh ginger, minced

2 Tbsp. Braggs Amino Acid

2 ½ Tbsp. rice wine vinegar

½ cup sesame oil

¼ cup extra-virgin olive oil

Salad Ingredients:

1 Tbsp. olive oil

1 cup shiitake mushrooms, sliced into ¼ inch pieces

1 cup shelled edamame beans

4 cups baby spinach leaves, washed and stemmed

½ cup cilantro leaves, roughly chopped

¼ cup unsalted dry roasted cashews

In a small saucepan, combine all vinaigrette ingredients and simmer over medium-low heat for 5 minutes. Set aside.

Prepare salad: Heat a large sauté pan over medium heat, and add oil and mushrooms, then sauté until cooked throughout. Add edamame and sauté to heat through, about 2 minutes. Add spinach and quickly heat until leaves just begin to wilt, about 1 minute.

Pour spinach mixture into a large mixing bowl and add cilantro and cashews. Season to taste with salt and pepper. Toss with just enough vinaigrette to coat and serve immediately.

SERVES

6

Colorful Slaw

INGREDIENTS

1 ½ cups fresh chickpeas

Olive oil cooking spray

4 tsp. extra virgin olive oil, divided

1 head broccoli stalks, shredded

1 head cabbage, shredded

1 head purple cabbage, shredded

1 ½ cup shelled edamame beans

¾ cup green or red bell pepper, julienned

1 ½ cup carrots, shredded

4 green onions, chopped

2/3 cup apple cider vinegar

2 Tbsp. raw organic honey

3 cloves garlic, minced

½ tsp. whole caraway seeds

½ tsp. fresh ground black pepper

Preheat oven to 450 degrees. Place chickpeas on a large roasting pan coated with cooking spray, and drizzle with 2 tsp. oil. Bake for 30 minutes, tossing occasionally. Remove from oven and let cool.

Combine broccoli, cabbages, edamame, bell pepper, carrots, and onions in a large bowl; set aside.

In a small bowl, whisk together vinegar, honey, garlic, caraway seeds, black pepper, and remaining 2 tsp. oil; pour over slaw, tossing gently. Chill for at least 30 minutes. Top with roasted chickpeas.

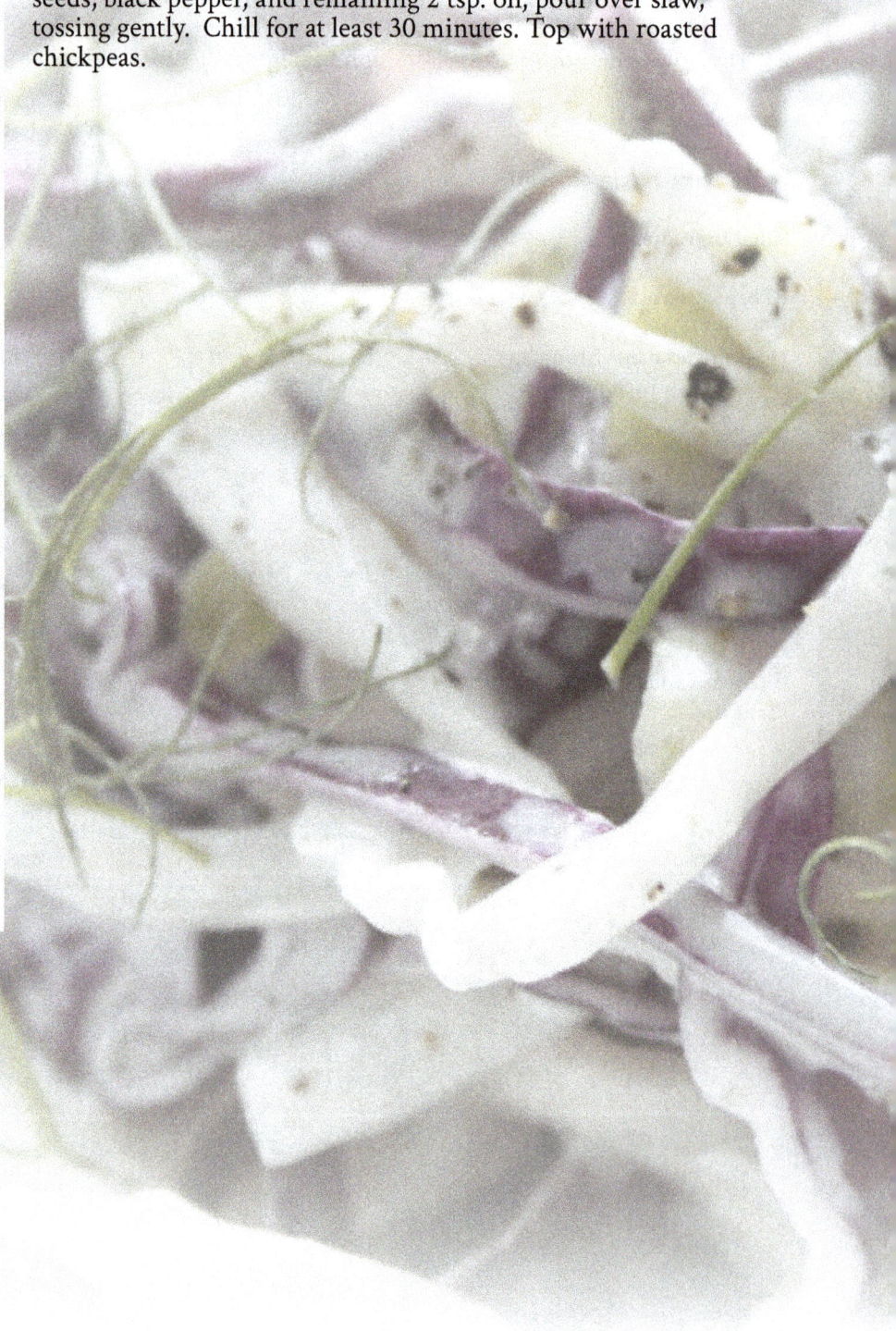

Apple Tangerine Greens

INGREDIENTS

1 (10 oz.) package baby greens

¼ cup red onion, chopped

½ cup walnuts, chopped

1/3 cup fat-free/reduced-fat crumbled blue cheese

2 ½ tsp. lemon zest

1 apple, peeled, cored, and sliced

1 avocado, peeled, pitted, and diced

4 mandarin oranges, juiced

½ lemon, juiced

½ tsp. lemon zest

2 clove garlic, minced

2 Tbsp. extra virgin olive oil

Salt to taste

In a large bowl, toss together the baby greens, red onion, walnuts, blue cheese, and lemon zest. Mix in the apple and avocado just before serving.

In a container with a lid, mix the mandarin orange juice, lemon juice, lemon zest, garlic, and olive oil.

Drizzle over the salad as desired.

SERVES

10

Sustaining your body with the proper nutrition is absolutely vital to achieving and maintaining optimal health. It is important to support healing and not contribute to degeneration. As you make the necessary changes to your diet, you will feel the difference good nutrition brings and we hope that these lifestyle alterations become permanent.

JR's Power Salad

INGREDIENTS

2 cups Romaine Lettuce

1 cup Fat Free Cottage Cheese

2 Tbsp. hummus (flavor of your choice)

4 oz. chicken

¼ cup fat-free Cheese

Mix all ingredients together.

Fresh Summer Salad

INGREDIENTS

2 Tbsp. extra-virgin olive oil

1 ½ Tbsp. balsamic vinegar

¼ tsp. freshly ground pepper

1 heart of romaine lettuce, torn or cut into bite-sized pieces (3 cups lightly packed)

1-8-oz container of strawberries, sliced

3 oz. (¾ cup) fat-free mozzarella cheese, diced

¼ cup fresh basil leaves, cut into ribbons

In a small bowl, whisk together oil, vinegar, and pepper. Place lettuce in a large bowl and toss with half of dressing. Place lettuce onto 4 salad plates.

Toss strawberries with remaining dressing and place ¼ of berries on top of each mound of lettuce.

Top each with cheese, and then sprinkle with basil.

Fancy Salad

INGREDIENTS

3 pieces pancetta, roughly chopped

2 tablespoons pine nuts

1 (12 ounce) package mixed baby salad greens

½ cucumber, halved, diced 1/2 –inch pieces

1 large tomato, diced in 1/2-inch pieces

12 kalamata olives, pitted and sliced in ½ vertically

2 tablespoons crumbled Gorgonzola

Freshly cracked black pepper

Dressing Ingredients:

2 cups loosely packed basil leaves

¾ cup balsamic vinegar

1 clove garlic put through garlic press

1 tablespoon Dijon mustard

½ teaspoon salt

½ cup extra-virgin olive oil

In a medium fry pan over medium heat, cook the pancetta until crispy. Remove to paper-towel lined plate to drain and cool. Clean out pan with paper towel and in same pan over medium heat, lightly toast the pine nuts. Remove to a plate and set aside to cool. Wash and dry greens, place in refrigerator to chill 10-15 minutes. Also chill individual salad plates or a platter if serving salad family-style.

When ready to serve, in a large bowl toss together salad greens, cucumber, and tomato with just enough dressing to lightly coat salad. Place salad on chilled individual plates or platter. Dress top of salad with pancetta, pine nuts, olives, Gorgonzola, and freshly cracked black pepper. Serve immediately.

Method for Dressing:

In a blender combine all ingredients except olive oil. Pulse several times until well combined. Once combined, turn machine on and slowly add in olive oil. Chill until ready to use.

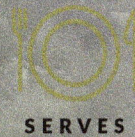

SERVES

6

Fresh Summer Salad

INGREDIENTS

2 Tbsp. extra-virgin olive oil

1 ½ Tbsp. balsamic vinegar

¼ tsp. freshly ground pepper

1 heart of romaine lettuce, torn or cut into bite-sized pieces (3 cups lightly packed)

1-8-oz container of strawberries, sliced

3 oz. (¾ cup) fat-free mozzarella cheese, diced

¼ cup fresh basil leaves, cut into ribbons

In a small bowl, whisk together oil, vinegar, and pepper. Place lettuce in a large bowl and toss with half of dressing. Place lettuce onto 4 salad plates.

Toss strawberries with remaining dressing and place ¼ of berries on top of each mound of lettuce.

Top each with cheese, and then sprinkle with basil.

SERVES

6

Caesar Salad

INGREDIENTS

Olive oil cooking spray

4 large garlic cloves, 3 of them chopped

4 slices Ezekiel Bread

4 boneless, skinless chicken breasts, about 1 ½ lb.

1 cup fat-free Greek yogurt

1 ½ Tbsp. Dijon mustard

Juice and zest of 2 lemons

2 ½ Tbsp. grated fat-free/reduced-fat Romano cheese

1 large head romaine, cleaned and cut into bite-size pieces

Preheat oven to 350 degrees. Place bread on a baking sheet and bake until golden brown and very crisp, about 8 minutes. Lightly bruise 1 whole garlic clove and rub it over the surface of each piece of bread. Cut bread into 1-inch cubes and set aside.

Meanwhile, preheat a grill or grill pan over high heat. Season chicken breasts with sea salt and pepper and spray lightly with cooking spray. Grill about 4 minutes per side, or until charred on the outside and just cooked through. Remove from grill and keep warm. Slice.

Meanwhile, together the 3 chopped garlic cloves with the Greek yogurt, Dijon mustard, lemon juice and zest, and cheese.

To serve toss together the romaine with the sliced chicken, dressing, and croutons. Adjust seasoning, if necessary.

SERVES

4

Yum-Yum Salad

INGREDIENTS

½ cup water

¼ cup quinoa

4 oz. lean turkey sausage
(or any lean sausage of your
choice)

1 ½ cup apples, diced

¼ cup walnuts, crushed

3 ½ cups fresh spinach

Bring water to a boil in a small pot on high heat. Add quinoa. Reduce heat to medium-low and cook for 12 minutes. Removed from heat, drain, and set aside to cool.

Cook sausage in a large pot of simmering water for 10 to 20 minutes, depending on the thickness.

Remove from water and preheat a nonstick pan on medium heat. Lightly coat with spray and add sausage. Sauté sausage until lightly browned all around. Set aside to cool. Then slice into medallions.

Combine all ingredients in a large mixing bowl. Drizzle your favorite dressing on the salad ("Sweet

Apple Vinaigrette with a Kick" is best, see page 69) and serve.

SERVES

2

Tropical Chicken Salad

INGREDIENTS

¼ cup fat-free yogurt

Juice from ½ lime

1 tsp. curry powder

½-15-oz can mixed tropical
fruit packed in juice,
unsweetened, drained

1 reserved cooked chicken
breast, diced into 1" pieces

1 bag pre-washed mixed
greens

In a small bowl, stir together yogurt, lime juice, and curry powder.

Place tropical fruit and chicken breast in a medium mixing bowl. Add yogurt dressing and stir to coat.

Divide mixed greens between 4 plates and top each with chicken salad.

SERVES

4

Thai Chicken Salad with Peanut Dressing

INGREDIENTS

¼ cup rice vinegar

2 Tbsp. natural smooth peanut butter

2 Tbsp. fresh ginger, chopped

2 tsp. chipotle pepper puree

1 ½ Tbsp. Braggs Amino Acid

1 Tbsp. honey

2 tsp. toasted sesame oil

½ cup extra-virgin olive oil

½ head Napa cabbage, shredded

½ head romaine lettuce, shredded

2 carrots, shredded

¼ lb snow peas, julienned

¼ cup coarsely chopped fresh cilantro leaves

¼ cup thinly sliced green onions

2 ¼ cups rotisserie chicken, shredded

½ cup roasted peanuts, chopped

¼ cup fresh mint leaves, chopped

Chili oil (optional)

Grilled lime halves, for garnish

Whisk together the vinegar, peanut butter, ginger, chipotle pepper puree, Braggs, honey, sesame oil, and olive oil in a medium bowl. Season with salt and pepper, to taste. Combine cabbage, lettuce, carrots, snow peas, cilantro, and green onion in a large bowl. Add the dressing and toss to combine.

Transfer to a serving platter and top with the shredded chicken, chopped peanuts, and mint. Drizzle with chili oil, if desired. Garnish with grilled lime halves.

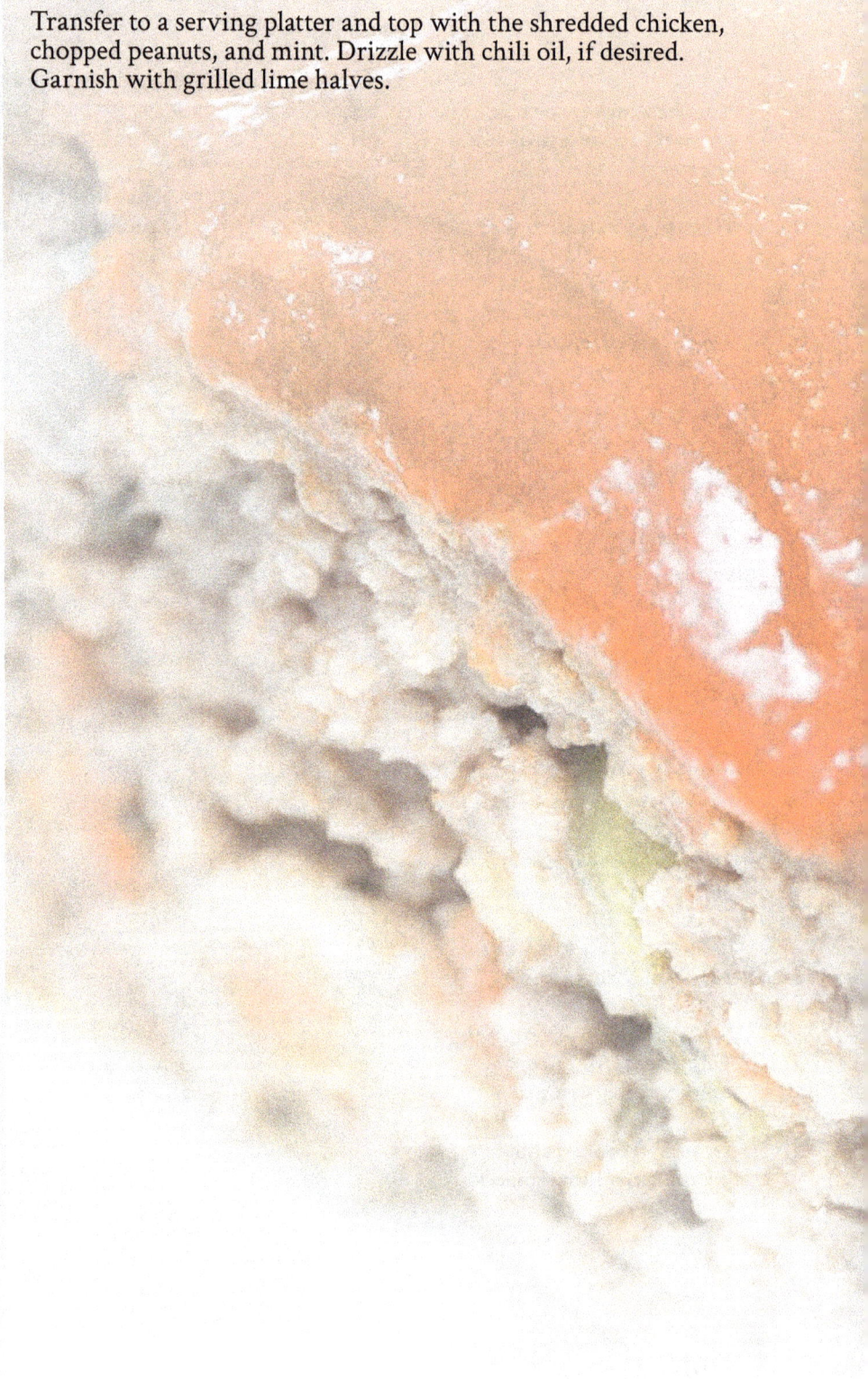

Spicy Beef Salad

INGREDIENTS

½ cup fresh lime juice

¼ cup bunch fresh cilantro, chopped and de-steamed

3 ½ Tbsp. sweet chili sauce

2 Tbsp. cloves minced garlic

1 ½ lb. lean flank steak, trimmed

Olive oil cooking spray

1 ¼ cup medium red onion, chopped

3 medium tomatoes, each cut into 6 wedges

6 cups romaine lettuce

1 ¼ cups cucumber, thinly sliced

2 Tbsp. fresh mint, chopped

2 Tbsp. unsalted raw peanuts (optional)

Preheat grill to medium-high heat or preheat broiler.

Combine first 4 ingredients in a small bowl, stirring well. Set half of lime mixture aside. Combine other half of lime mixture with steak in a large zip-top plastic bag and seal. Marinate in refrigerator for 20 minutes, turning once. Remove steak from bag and discard marinade.

Place steak on grill rack or broiler pan coated with cooking spray and cook 6 minutes per side for medium or until it reaches desired doneness. Let stand 5 minutes. Cut steak diagonally, across grain, into thin slices.

Heat a large nonstick skillet coated with cooking spray over medium-high heat. Add onion and sauté for 3 minutes. Add tomatoes and sauté for 2 more minutes. Place onion-tomato mixture, lettuce, cucumber, and mint in a large bowl; toss gently to combine. Divide salad evenly and top each serving with 3 oz. steak. Drizzle each salad with 1 tablespoon reserved lime mixture and sprinkle with peanuts, if desired.

SERVES

8

4 Quarter Protein Balls

INGREDIENTS

2 ¾ cups dates, seeds removed

½ cup water

¾ cup natural peanut butter

1 cup whey protein powder

¼ cup unsweetened, non-dutched (unprocessed) cocoa

1/8 cup ground flaxseeds

2 tsp. cinnamon

2 Tbsp. sesame seeds

½ cup ground walnuts or almonds

In a food processor, blend dates and water. Add peanut butter and blend until smooth. Add protein powder in ½ cup increments and process. Then mix in cocoa, flaxseeds, cinnamon, and sesame seeds.

With clean hands gather some dough (about the size of a golf ball) and roll it between the palms of your hands. Keep a bowl of protein powder nearby, if dough becomes sticky, roll it in the protein powder to keep it from sticking to your hands. (Note: Refrigerating the dough overnight makes it easier to work with the next day).

Roll each ball in the ground walnuts. Set each ball on a baking sheet. Place in the freezer for 2 to 4 hours. Serve or freeze for later.

SERVES

12

West Clinic Approved Protein Bars

INGREDIENTS

2 cups Peanut Butter

¾ cup honey or agave nectar

1 ¾ cups protein (about 7 scoops Whey Protein), any protein flavor, but vanilla tastes the best

2 cups old-fashion oats

2 Tbsp. cinnamon

1/3 cup almond slivers

In a bowl combine dry ingredients: protein, oats, cinnamon, and almonds.

In another bowl (glass bowl) combine peanut butter and honey and microwave for 1 minute, then stir.

Combine directions 1 and 2, place in a pan (with wax paper at the bottom of pan) and cut in 20 equal bars.

Gluten Free Meatloaf

INGREDIENTS

1 lb. lean ground turkey or chicken or any lean ground meat

1 cup cooked brown rice

1 egg

¾ cup plain, fat-free yogurt cheese (refer to page 76)

½ cup onion, finely chopped

½ cup red, green, or yellow bell peppers, finely chopped

½ cup celery, finely chopped

1 Tbsp. tamari

Fresh ground black pepper

1 ½ tsp. crumbled dried oregano

2 tsp. crumbled dried basil

Cooking spray

Preheat oven to 350 degrees.

In a large mixing bowl combine all ingredients with a pair of clean hands. Place in a loaf pan that has been prepared with a light coating of nonstick cooking spray. Bake for about an hour. Remove from oven and let stand for 10 minutes before cutting.

SERVES

6

Turkey Meatloaf

INGREDIENTS

1 small yellow onion, coarsely chopped

1 medium carrot, peeled and coarsely chopped

1 stalk of celery coarsely chopped

2 canned chipotle peppers in adobo sauce

1 (20 oz.) package extra-lean ground turkey breast

½ cup quick cooking oats

2 eggs whites

½ pepper, color of your choice

Ingredients for Topping:

¼ cup no high-fructose corn syrup, no sugar added ketchup

2 Tbsp. chipotle pepper adobo sauce

1 Tbsp. Stevia

Preheat oven to 350 degrees. In the work bowl of a food processor, combine onion, carrots, celery, and pepper. Pulse until finely chopped. Add chipotle pepper sauce and pulse until just combined. In a large bowl, combine the ground turkey with the pepper and vegetable mixture. Add egg whites and oats; gently mix until combined. Place about 1/3 cup of the prepared meatloaf mixture into 9 wells of a standard size muffin pan that has been lightly sprayed with nonstick cooking spray. Bake for 20 minutes.

Meanwhile, combine all the topping ingredients in a small bowl; set aside. Remove meat loaves from oven and spoon the topping over each meatloaf. Return meatloaf to the oven and continue to bake for an additional 5 to 10 minutes or until meatloaf is firm and the internal temperature registers 165*.

Let meatloaf stand for 5 minutes before serving.

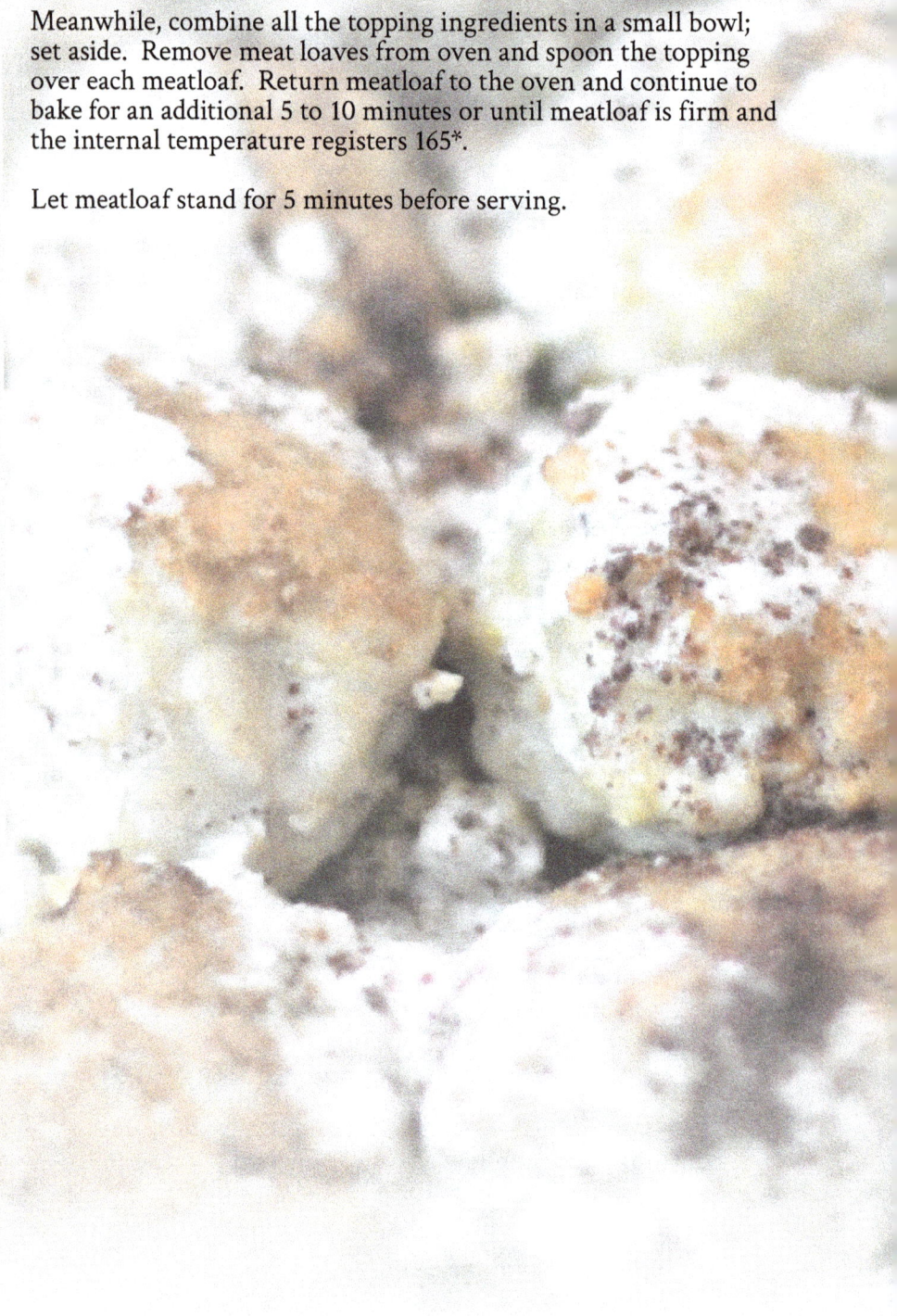

Marinara Turkey Meatballs

INGREDIENTS

3 lbs ground turkey

2 cups cooked quinoa

½ onion, chopped

3 large eggs

3 Tbsp. Italian parsley

1 cup grated parmesan cheese

3 Tbsp. olive oil (divided)

Marinara Sauce Ingredients:

3 28oz cans diced tomatoes

3 cloves garlic, minced

2 Tbsp. olive oil

1 Tbsp. dried oregano

Ground pepper to taste

In a skillet, sauté onion and garlic in 1 Tbsp. of olive oil for about 5 minutes over medium heat (for meatballs). Set aside to cool to room temperature.

In a large sauce pan, heat olive oil and garlic for about 5 minutes. Add the tomatoes and oregano and bring to a boil. Lower to a simmer and continue to cook for 30 minutes. Add ground pepper to taste.

In a large bowl combine ground turkey, cooked quinoa, sautéed onion and garlic, 3 eggs, parmesan cheese, and parsley. Use your hands to mix everything together. Shape meat into balls.

In a large skillet, cook meatballs in remaining olive oil. Cook until meatballs are brown on the bottom and then flip them over to cook until brown on that side. (Will need to be done in batches rather than all at once). Remove meatballs and place them on a paper towel-lined plate to remove excess oil.

After marinara has cooked for 30 minutes, add cooked meatballs and let simmer for about 45 minutes.

Greek Chicken Breast with Cucumber Yogurt Sauce

INGREDIENTS

¼ tsp. cumin seeds

¼ tsp. fennel seeds

¼ tsp. coriander seeds

1 tsp. cayenne pepper

¼ tsp. turmeric powder

¼ cup Greek Yogurt

2 boneless, skinless chicken breasts

2 tsp. lemon juice

1 tsp. garlic, minced

½ cucumber, peeled and finely diced

4 cups mixed baby salad greens

¼ cup fresh cilantro

Preheat a grill or grill pan.

Place a small sauté pan over medium-high heat and toast each of the seeds separately for 1 to 2 minutes and remove from pan to a mixing bowl to cool.

Using a mortar and pestle or a food processor grind the spices into a powder being sure to break up any large pieces of the seeds.

Pass the spice mix through a small sifter into a mixing bowl and mix well, set aside.

On a clean work surface lay out several even layers of plastic wrap and place on chicken breast over the plastic. Cover the chicken with another piece of layered plastic and lightly pound the chicken breast with a meat mallet or meat tenderizer until the chicken breast is thinned out to about a ½ inch thickness. Repeat with the second chicken breast.

Lightly brush the grill with a little olive oil. Season each side of the chicken generously with the spice mix and reserve any remaining spice mix for a later use in an airtight container. Place the chicken breasts on the grill and cook for 3 to 4 minutes on each side or until an instant read thermometer inserted into the chicken reads 165 degrees.

While the chicken is cooking, mix the lemon juice, garlic, cucumber, and yogurt in a small mixing bowl until well incorporated.

Remove the chicken from the grill to a plate and let rest for 2 to 3 minutes. Arrange the greens on a large serving platter. Place the chicken breasts atop the greens and drizzle the sauce over and around the chicken. Garnish the chicken with cilantro leaves and serve.

101

SERVES

4

Cajun Jambalaya

INGREDIENTS

14 oz. boneless, skinless chicken breast, diced

1 red onion, diced

½ tsp. garlic, minced

14 oz. can no salt added tomatoes with juice, chopped

1 red pepper, diced

1 yellow pepper, diced

½ cup frozen corn kernels

2 tsp. hot sauce

2 tsp. chili powder

½ tsp. dried oregano

Fresh ground pepper

2 ½ cup low-sodium chicken stock

1 ½ cup brown rice

¾ cup frozen peas

1 tsp. paprika

3 ½ Tbsp. parsley, chopped

½ tsp. red pepper flakes

Put chicken, onion, garlic, chicken stock, tomatoes with juice, and rice into a large pan. Add the chili powder, paprika, oregano, and red pepper flakes, and stir well. Bring to a boil then reduce heat, cover, and let simmer for 25 minutes.

Add the peppers, corn, and peas to the rice mixture and return to a boil. Reduce heat, cover, and let simmer for an additional 10 minutes until rice is tender.

Stir 2 Tbsp. of parsley and season to taste with pepper. Garnish with remaining parsley.

SERVES

4

Balsamic Chicken Sautee

INGREDIENTS

¼ cup whole wheat flour

4 boneless, skinless chicken breasts halves

2 Tbsp. extra-virgin olive oil

2 cups red onion, sliced long and thin

1 cup low-sodium chicken broth

2 Tbsp. balsamic vinegar

1 teaspoon dried thyme leaves

½ tsp. dried basil leaves

Mix flour and chicken; turn to coat. Shake off excess.

Heat oil in a large cast-iron or other heavy skillet over medium heat. Add chicken and cook, turning once, 10 minutes or until browned and cooked through. Remove to a plate to keep warm.

Add onion to skillet and sauté 1 to 2 minutes until lightly browned. Add broth, vinegar, thyme, and basil. Bring to a boil and cook, stirring often, 7 minutes or until onions are soft and sauce is syrupy. Then spoon over chicken.

SERVES

4

It is **important** to keep your motivation up while striving to eat healthy. It will be challenging, especially in the beginning weeks. Stay focused on your goal - attaining optimal health and healing.

Party Ready Chicken Breasts

INGREDIENTS

2 lb. boneless, skinless chicken breasts

2 Tbsp. extra-virgin olive oil

3 tsp. dried rosemary

10 large leaves fresh sage

1 ½ cups dry red wine

4 tsp. garlic, minced

½ tsp. red pepper flakes

Garnish: fresh sage cut in narrow strips

Season chicken with pepper. Heat oil in a large heavy nonstick skillet over medium heat. Add chicken, rosemary, and sage and cook, turning chicken occasionally, 15 minutes or until golden brown.

Add ¼ cup of the wine, the garlic, and pepper flakes.

Cook 20 minutes longer, turning chicken occasionally and spooning on all but 2 Tbsp. of the wine as pan juices evaporate, until chicken is cooked through and coated with a deep brown blaze. Remove to warm serving plates.

Add remaining 2 Tbsp. wine to skillet and cook, stirring in browned drippings from bottom of pan.

Spoon pan juices over chicken and garnish.

SERVES

4

Glazed Chicken

INGREDIENTS

Juice of 3 oranges

1 Tbsp. Dijon mustard

1 Tbsp. honey or Stevia

1 tsp. garlic, minced

1 Tbsp. fresh ginger, finely chopped

4 boneless, skinless chicken breasts, cubed

6 large sprigs of rosemary with half the leaves removed

Garnish: an orange sliced evenly

Preheat a grill or grill pan on medium-high heat.

Place the orange juice into a small saucepan and cook over medium heat until the orange juice has the consistency of a very thin syrup.

Add the Dijon mustard, honey/Stevia, garlic, and ginger and continue cooking over medium heat for 2 to 3 minutes.

Remove from heat to allow flavors to blend and reserve.

Evenly divide the cubed chicken among the rosemary sprigs and skewer the chicken onto the exposed part of the rosemary sprigs.

Lightly brush the grill with oil and grill chicken for 1 to 2 minutes on each side or until the internal temperature of the chicken reaches 165 degrees on an instant read thermometer.

Remove skewers from the grill to a serving plate, drizzle with the orange sauce and serve immediately.

Health-A-Fried Chicken

INGREDIENTS

4-7 oz. boneless, skinless chicken breasts

1 ½ cups fat-free buttermilk or almond or rice milk

Olive oil cooking spray

2 tsp. dry mustard

1 tsp. onion powder

½ tsp. garlic powder

½ tsp. ground black pepper

1 tsp. cayenne pepper

1 cup 100% whole wheat panko

1 Tbsp. parsley

Place chicken breasts in a re-sealable plastic container that is slightly larger than the breasts. Pour buttermilk or whatever milk you decide to use, over breasts, then turn them so they are completely coated. Let marinate in refrigerator for at least 6 hours or overnight, rotating them once or twice.

Preheat oven to 450 degrees. Lightly mist a medium, nonstick baking sheet with spray.

In a small bowl, mix mustard, onion powder, garlic powder, black pepper, and cayenne.

Add panko to a medium, shallow bowl.

Remove 1 chicken breast from buttermilk, allowing any excess liquid to drip off. Sprinkle both sides of breast evenly with ¼ of seasoning mixture. Then transfer it to bowl of panko and parsley, covering it completely with crumbs. Place breaded chicken breast face down on prepared pan. Repeat with remaining chicken breasts.

Lightly mist top of breasts with spray. Bake chicken for 10 minutes, then gently, being careful not to remove any breading, flip the breasts. Lightly mist them again with spray and continue to bake for another 10 to 15 minutes or until breading is crispy and chicken is no longer pink inside. Serve immediately or refrigerate for up to 2 days to eat cold.

Crispy Chicken Fingers

INGREDIENTS

12 ounces skinless, boneless chicken breast halves

1 egg, slightly beaten

1 Tbsp. organic raw honey, Stevia, or agave nectar

1 tsp. prepared mustard

2 cups 100% whole wheat flakes, finely crushed

4 Tbsp. 100% whole wheat panko

1 tsp. ground pepper

Preheat oven to 450 degrees. Cut chicken into 3-by-3/4-inch strips. In a shallow dish, combine egg, honey, and mustard. In another dish, stir together flake crumbs, panko, and pepper.

Dip chicken strips into the egg mixture; roll in crumb mixture to coat. Arrange chicken strips on an ungreased baking sheet.

Bake about 12 minutes, or until outsides are golden and chicken is no longer pink.

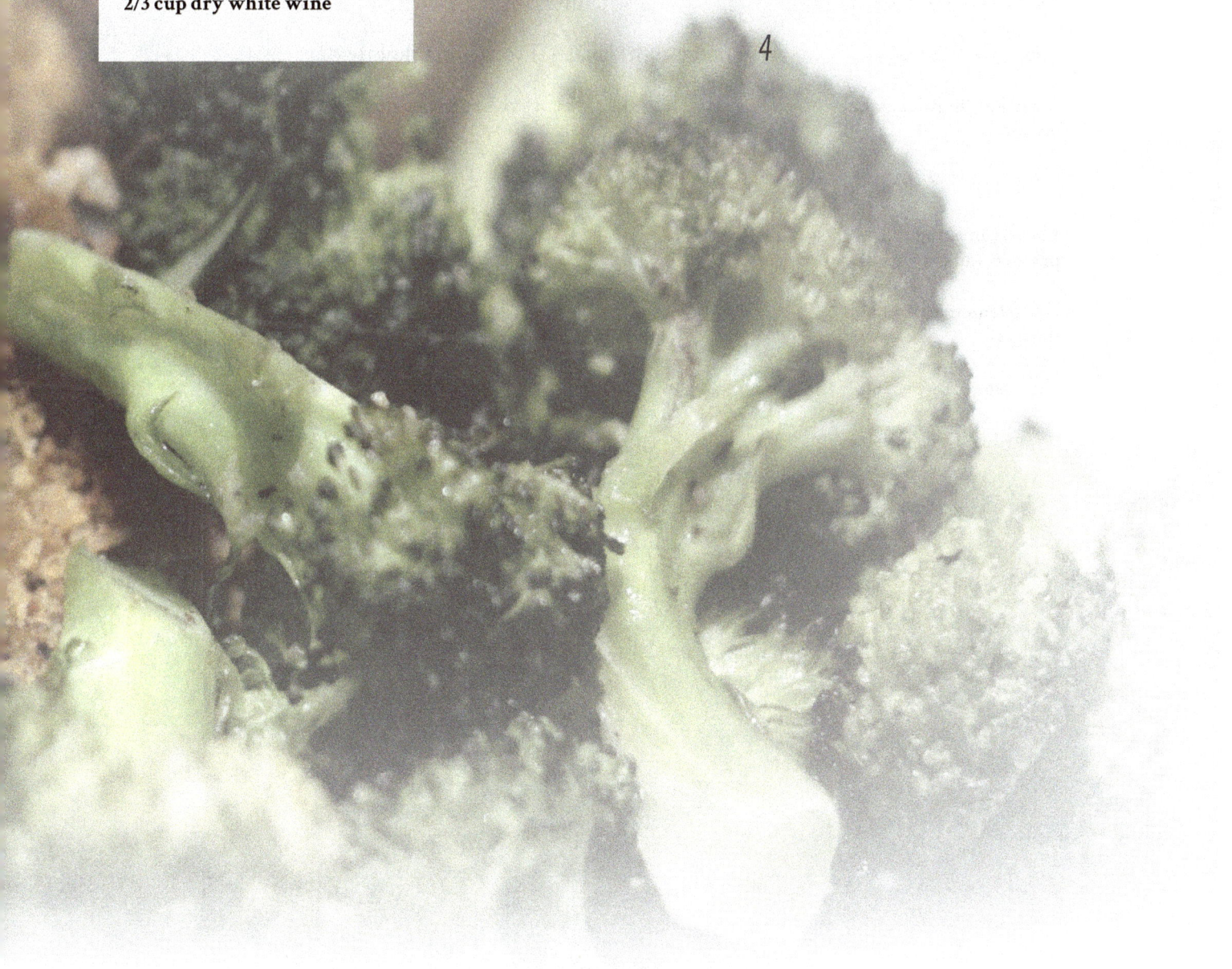

Simple Chicken

INGREDIENTS

4 boneless, skinless chicken breasts

1 ½ Tbsp. fresh rosemary leaves, chopped

1 tsp. grated lemon zest

2 tsp. lemon juice

Olive oil cooking spray

2/3 cup dry white wine

Combine rosemary, zest, and pepper in a small cup; rub mixture over chicken.

Spray a large nonstick skillet with cooking spray and place over medium heat. Add chicken and cook for 5 minutes. Place a heavy cast-iron skillet over chicken and continue to cook 10 to 12 minutes, or until skin is crisp and chicken is cooked through.

Transfer chicken to plates. Pour wine and lemon juice into skillet, raise heat to high, and boil 2 minutes, scraping up browned bits from bottom of skillet with a wooden spoon; spoon over chicken.

SERVES

4

Lemon Chicken

INGREDIENTS

¼ cup 100% whole wheat flour

1 Tbsp. dried oregano

1 lb. boneless, skinless thin chicken cutlet

Olive oil cooking spray

½ Tbsp. extra-virgin olive oil

1 yellow onion, thinly sliced

1 tsp. garlic, minced

¼ cup low-sodium chicken broth

¼ cup peas

1-14 oz. can artichoke hearts, drained and cut into sixths

¼ cup lemon juice (about 2 lemons)

2 tsp. lemon zest

Garnish: 2 Tbsp. parsley

In a shallow bowl, thoroughly combine flour, oregano, and pepper. Dredge each chicken cutlet in flour mixture, shake off excess and place on a plate.

Coat a large nonstick skillet with cooking spray and heat on medium to medium-high, so skillet is hot but not smoking. Add ½ the chicken cutlets and cook 3 to 5 minutes per side, until lightly browned and cooked through. Transfer to a clean serving plate and repeat with remaining cutlets, coating skillet once more with cooking spray. Cover your serving plate with foil to keep chicken warm.

Adjust temperature to medium-low and heat oil. Place onion in pan and cook. Stir frequently until soft and golden, 5 to 6 minutes. Add garlic, cooking for 1 minute, stirring constantly; then chicken broth, bringing it to a simmer; followed by artichokes, peas, lemon juice, and zest, simmering for 2 to

minutes until heated through and slightly thickened.

Pour artichoke mixture over chicken cutlets, sprinkle with parsley and serve.

SERVES

4

French Chicken

INGREDIENTS

2 tsp. extra-virgin olive oil

4 boneless, skinless chicken breast

1 cup onion, sliced thin

1 tsp. garlic, finely chopped

1 red bell pepper, diced

2 cups button mushrooms, diced

¼ cup red wine

2 cups sodium-free fire roasted tomatoes

1 cup Roma tomatoes

1 sprig thyme

1 bay leaf

1 tsp. dried oregano

1 cup broccoli, cut into small pieces

1 Tbsp. parsley, chopped

5 kalamata olives, chopped

1 cup steamed brown rice to serve

Heat a large saucepot over medium-high heat and add 1 tsp. oil to the pan.

Season the chicken with pepper and sear for 2 to 3 minutes on each side or until golden brown.

Remove the chicken to a plate and add the remaining oil to the pan.

Sauté the onions for 3 minutes stirring constantly. Then add the garlic and bell peppers.

Cook the garlic and peppers for 2 minutes and add the mushrooms.

Cook the mushrooms for 4 minutes stirring often.

Add the red wine and reduce until almost dry.

Add the tomatoes to the pot and stir well.

Add the thyme, bay leaf, and oregano.

Bring to the simmer and reduce heat to low.

Add the chicken back to the sauce and simmer gently for 8 to 10 minutes or until the chicken is cooked through and the sauce has thickened slightly.

Stir in all but one pinch of the parsley.

To serve, spoon ¼ cup of brown rice onto the center of a serving plate.

Place on portion of chicken on top of the rice and spoon some of the sauce and vegetables over the chicken, repeat with remaining plates.

Sprinkle a little of the chopped olives and remaining parsley over each plate of chicken and serve.

SERVES

4

Power Chicken with Spicy Peanut Sauce

INGREDIENTS

½ cup low-sodium chicken broth

½ cup unsweetened light coconut milk

2 Tbsp. Braggs Amino Acid or tamari sauce

1 shallot, thinly sliced

1 tsp. garlic, minced

2 tsp. Asian fish sauce

1 Tbsp. Stevia

½ tsp. finely grated lime zest

2 Tbsp. ginger, minced

1 lb. skinless, boneless chicken breast halves, pounded slightly between 2 sheets of waxed paper and cut across into 1-inch-thick strips

Olive oil cooking spray

Eight 8-inch bamboo skewers, soaked in water for 20 minutes

3 Tbsp. fresh basil, minced

4 Tbsp. cilantro, minced

¼ cup unsalted peanuts, chopped

In a medium bowl, whisk together the broth, coconut milk, soy sauce, shallot, garlic, fish sauce, Stevia, lime zest, and ginger. Add the chicken strips, toss to coat them evenly, cover with plastic wrap, and marinate in the refrigerator for 1 hour.

Remove the chicken from the marinade and discard the marinade.

Coat a nonstick grill pan with cooking spray and set it over medium-high heat. While the pan is heating, thread the chicken onto the skewers. Place the skewers in the hot pan and sear until cooked through and the chicken has light grill marks, 2 to 3 minutes per side.

Serve the chicken skewers garnished with the basil, cilantro, and chopped peanuts.

SERVES

4

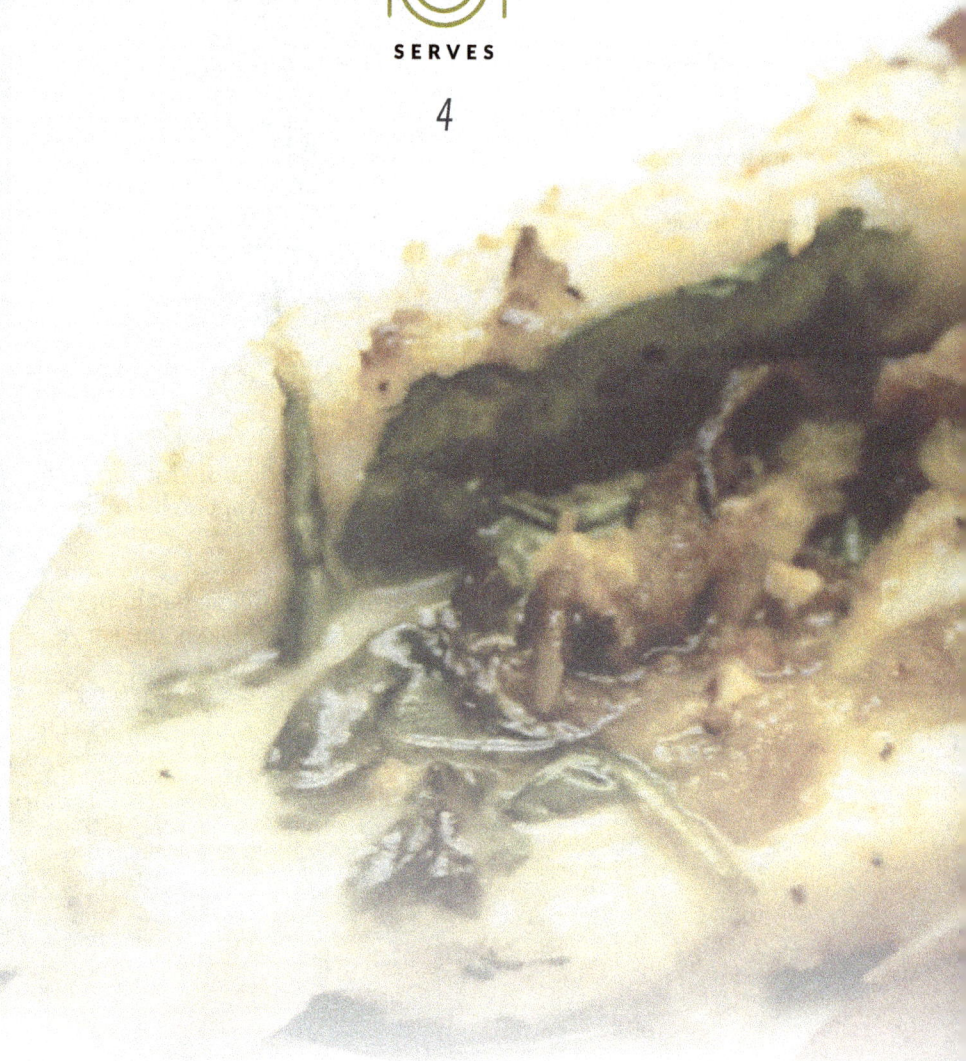

Stuffed Chicken Breast Party Stoppers

INGREDIENTS

1 cup strawberries, chopped

½ cup Stevia

½ cup sherry vinegar

1/3 cup less-sodium chicken broth

¼ tsp. ground coriander

Ground black pepper, to taste

1 tsp. parsley

Chicken Ingredients:

¼ cup crumbled Gorgonzola cheese

3 tsp. fresh thyme leaves

2 oz. prosciutto, chopped

4 skinless, boneless chicken breast halves

Olive oil cooking spray

1/8 teaspoon freshly ground black pepper

To prepare sauce, place strawberries in a small, heavy saucepan; partially mash with a fork. Stir in sweetener, vinegar, broth, coriander, black pepper, and parsley; bring to a boil. Reduce heat, and simmer until reduced to 2/3 cup (about 30 minutes), stirring occasionally. Strain mixture through a sieve over a bowl; discard solids.

To prepare chicken, combine cheese, thyme, and prosciutto in a bowl. Cut a horizontal slit through thickest portion of each chicken breast half to form a pocket; spoon 3 Tbsp. cheese mixture into each pocket.

Heat a large nonstick skillet over medium heat. Coat pan with cooking spray. Sprinkle both sides of chicken evenly with pepper. Add chicken to pan; cook 5 minutes or until browned. Turn chicken over; cook 4 minutes or until done. Serve with sauce.

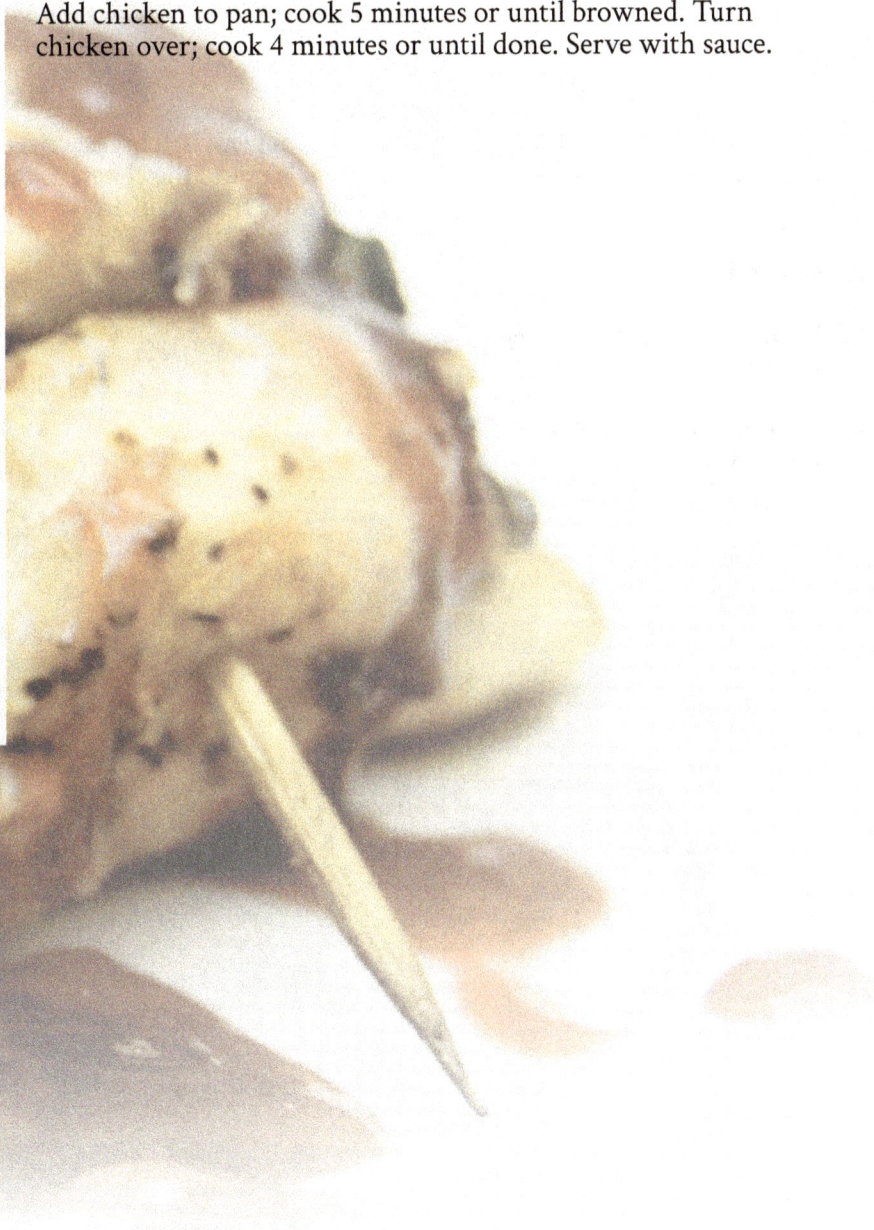

Stuffed Chicken Bake

INGREDIENTS

2 Tbsp. extra-virgin olive oil

1 tsp. dried thyme

1 tsp. red pepper flakes

1 (7 oz.) jar artichoke hearts, drained, rinsed, chopped

1 tsp. garlic, minced

3 oz. fat-free feta cheese with herbs

3 Tbsp. oil-packed sun-dried tomatoes, drained, minced

2 Tbsp. fresh basil, finely chopped

¼ cup fresh dill, sprigs pulled off the steam

4 boneless, skinless chicken breasts halves

Rinse chicken breasts under cold water and pat dry. Place each breast between 2 sheets of plastic wrap and gently beat with mallet to flatten to ¼-inch.

Warm 1 Tbsp. olive oil, thyme, and red pepper flakes in a medium-sized sauté pan over medium-high heat for 1 to 2 minutes. Then add artichoke hearts, garlic, and pepper and cook for 3 to 4 minutes occasionally stirring.

Remove pan from heat, add feta cheese, sun-dried tomatoes, basil, and dill, then mix to evenly distribute ingredients and allow stuffing to cool.

Place breasts side down, and spread each one with ¼ of the stuffing. Fold the breasts in half over stuffing and use toothpicks to hold closed.

Brush each side of the chicken with remaining oil and season with garlic and pepper. Grill breasts over direct medium heat until meat juices run clear and the cheese is melted (8-12 minutes) turning once. Remove from grill and carefully remove toothpick.

SERVES
4

Thai Coconut Chicken

INGREDIENTS

1 cup brown jasmine rice

1-14 oz. can light coconut milk

1 cup low-sodium chicken broth

1 ½ Tbsp. cornstarch

1 Tbsp. ginger, minced

2 strips fresh lime peel

1 lb. boneless, skinless chicken breast, cut into strips

2 cups snow peas

1 Tbsp. low-sodium fish sauce

¼ cup cilantro leaves, chopped

Lime wedges

Prepare rice as label directs.

Meanwhile, in 12-inch nonstick skillet, stir together coconut milk, broth, cornstarch, ginger, and lime peel; heat to boiling over medium-high heat, stirring frequently. Boil for 1 minute.

Add chicken and snow peas to skillet; cover and cook 4 to 5 minutes longer or until chicken doesn't have the pink color throughout. Remove skillet from heat; stir in fish sauce and cilantro. Serve with rice and lime wedges.

SERVES

4

Buffalo Chicken with Gyro Sauce

INGREDIENTS

½ cup fat-free plain Greek yogurt

2 Tbsp. fat-free buttermilk

2 Tbsp. white wine vinegar

1/3 cup fat-free feta cheese, crumbled

¼ cup green onions, chopped

4 Tbsp. Frank's hot sauce

3 Tbsp. Frank's hot buffalo sauce

1 Tbsp. extra-virgin olive oil

1 Tbsp. paprika

4 boneless, skinless chicken breasts, each cut into 2, 3-inch pieces

Olive oil cooking spray

In a medium bowl, whisk together yogurt, buttermilk, vinegar, feta, and onions. Cover and refrigerate mixture until ready to serve or for up to 2 days.

In a small bowl, combine hot sauces, oil, and paprika. Place chicken in a large shallow dish. Pour hot sauce mixture over chicken, tossing to coat. Cover and marinate for at least 30 minutes at room temperature or in the refrigerator for up to 8 hours.

Preheat oven to 400 degrees. Mist a large baking sheet with cooking spray. Remove chicken from hot sauce marinade, discarding marinade, and place chicken on baking sheet. Bake for 8 to 10 minutes or until chicken is cooked through (no need to flip). Top with buttermilk-feta sauce, dividing evenly, or pour sauce into a separate bowl for dipping.

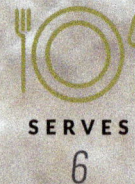

SERVES
6

Becoming educated and informed in my own nutrition has opened my eyes to a new and better way of healing - from the inside out!

-Kristine May

Pecan Pie Crusted Chicken

INGREDIENTS

½ cup pecan halves

2 slices whole wheat bread, torn into pieces

2 egg whites, lightly beaten

1 lb. boneless, skinless chicken breast tenders, 12 pieces total

¼ tsp. dried thyme

½ tsp. chives

1 Tbsp. + 1 tsp. extra-virgin olive oil

½ cup apricot or peach 100% fruit spread

1 lemon freshly squeezed of its juice

Preheat oven to 425 degrees. Coat a rimmed baking sheet with cooking spray.

Put pecans in food processor and chop. Add bread and pulse to fine crumbs. Transfer to shallow dish.

Put egg whites in another dish and beat lightly with the chives. Sprinkle chicken with thyme.

Dip a piece of chicken into egg whites and then roll in crumbs, pressing to adhere. Place on prepared baking sheet. Repeat with remaining chicken. Drizzle chicken with oil. Bake 12 to 15 minutes, until crumbs brown and chicken is no longer pink in thickest part.

Mix fruit spread and lemon juice in bowl to make sauce.

SERVES

4

Black and Blue Chicken Stuffed Potatoes

INGREDIENTS

6 russet potatoes, peel left on and scrubbed well

Olive oil cooking spray

½ lb (about 2 breasts) boneless, skinless chicken breasts, chopped

1 tsp. fresh ground black pepper

2 tsp. extra-virgin olive oil

2 cups baby spinach

¼ cup small yellow or red onion, chopped

¼ cup reduced-fat crumbled blue cheese

2 Tbsp. fat-free plain cream cheese

1 tsp. fresh lemon juice

Preheat oven to 400 degrees. With a fork, poke holes in potatoes. Wrap potatoes separately in foil and bake in a large baking dish misted with cooking spray for 45 minutes to 1 hour or until tender; let cool at least 15 minutes.

Season chicken with 1 tsp. pepper. Heat oil in a large skillet over medium-high heat. Add chicken and cook for 5 to 7 minutes or until cooked through; remove from skillet and set aside. Add spinach and onion to same skillet and sauté over medium heat until spinach is wilted. Remove from heat; set aside.

Cut potatoes in half lengthwise. Carefully scoop out centers, leaving ¼-inch-thick shells. In a large mixing bowl, mash potato meat; set aside.

Stir chicken and spinach mixture into potato meat. Add blue cheese, cream cheese, lemon juice, and stir well. Spoon mixture into potato shells, dividing evenly, and place potatoes, cut-side-up, on a baking sheet misted with cooking spray.

Bake for 10 to 15 minutes or until lightly browned and thoroughly heated.

SERVES

6

Sesame Chicken Stir-Fry

INGREDIENTS

2 tsp. sesame seeds

2 boneless, skinless chicken breast, cut in chucks

1 Tbsp. whole wheat flour

2 ½ tsp. extra-virgin olive oil

1 lb. bunch bok choy, stalks and leaves cut in half lengthwise, then in pieces crosswise, leaves and stalks separated

2 red peppers, cut in long strips

1/3 cup each stir-fry sauce, orange juice and water

2 tsp. grated orange zest

½ cup green onion

Cook sesame seeds in large nonstick skillet over medium heat until golden and fragrant. Set aside.

Put chicken and flour in Ziploc bag. Seal and shake to coat.

Heat 2 tsp. oil in same skillet until hot but not smoking. Add chicken; stir-fry 5 minutes until opaque in center. Remove to a large plate.

Heat remaining oil in skillet with bok choy stalks, peppers, and onions, cooking 5 minutes or until almost crisp-tender.

Add bok choy leaves; stir-fry 2 minutes. Mix remaining ingredients. Stir into skillet. Return chicken; stir until simmering. Place on serving plate; sprinkle with sesame seeds.

SERVES
4

Chicken Fried Rice

INGREDIENTS

1 Tbsp. + 1 tsp. extra-virgin olive oil

3 cups cooked brown rice

2 cans no salt added chicken breast

Low-sodium, gluten-free tamari sauce or Braggs Amino Acid

2 cups cooked vegetables

2 eggs + 3 egg whites

Heat olive oil in skillet over medium-high heat, add rice and brown. Then add vegetables until heated. Beat eggs and egg whites, make a clearing in the middle of the pan and scramble the eggs. Mix all together and add soy sauce to taste.

SERVES
4

Beef & Broccoli Asian Stir-Fry

INGREDIENTS

12 oz. soba noodles

Olive oil cooking spray

1 lb. lean round steak, sliced into strips

½ cup white onion, diced

2 cups fresh broccoli small florets pieces

½ red bell pepper, julienne cut

3 Tbsp. Braggs Amino Acid or tamari sauce

Juice of 1 medium orange

2 Tbsp. orange zest

1 tsp. garlic, minced

2 tsp. raw organic honey or Stevia

2 tsp. 100% whole wheat flour

Cook noodles according to package directions. Drain and set aside.

Heat large nonstick or cast-iron skillet over high heat for 1 minute. Reduce heat to medium-high, mist pan with cooking spray and sauté steak for about 5 minutes or until cooked through. (For medium doneness, the steak will still be slightly pink in the middle.) Remove steak, leaving juices in the pan.

Mist same pan again with cooking spray. Add onion, broccoli, and pepper and sauté over medium- high heat for about 5 minutes or until cooked through.

In a medium bowl, whisk together Braggs/tamari sauce, orange juice and zest, garlic, and honey/Stevia.

Add steak back to vegetables in pan and pour in soy sauce mixture. Sauté steak and vegetables over medium-high heat for about 2 minutes, then whisk in flour to thicken, about 2 to 3 minutes. Add noodles to pan and cook until warmed, about 3 more minutes. Remove from heat and serve.

Beef and Quinoa Stir Fry

INGREDIENTS

1 cup quinoa

1 Tbsp. olive oil

1 cup chopped onion

2 cloves garlic, minced

1 green bell pepper, chopped

1 orange bell pepper, chopped

1 red bell pepper, chopped

1 lb lean beef tenderloin, trim fat and cut into strips

1 cup low-sodium beef broth

¼ cup chopped basil

Ground pepper to taste

Cook quinoa according to package and set aside.

In a large wok or skillet, heat olive oil over medium-high heat. Add onions and garlic and cook for 2-3 minutes. Add bell peppers and cook for 2 more minutes. Add beef and cook for another 2 minutes. Add broth and let simmer for another 2 minutes or until steak is cooked through. Remove from heat

Add quinoa, basil, and ground pepper and mix well before serving

Pork Cutlets

INGREDIENTS

1 lb. pork tenderloin

¼ cup whole wheat flour

1 Tbsp. extra-virgin olive oil, divided

½ cup reduced-sodium chicken broth

½ cup white wine or reduced-sodium chicken broth

1 tsp. lemon juice

2 Tbsp. capers, drained

1 Tbsp. fresh parsley, minced

Cut pork into eight slices. In a large re-sealable plastic bag, combine the flour and add pork, one piece at a time, and shake to coat. In a large nonstick skillet cook over medium heat, cook pork in oil in batches for 2-3 minutes on each side or until juices run clear. Remove and keep warm.

Add broth, wine, and lemon juice to the pan, stirring to loosen browned bits. Stir in capers. Bring to a boil. Reduce heat; simmer, uncovered, for 4-6 minutes or until juices are slightly thickened. Stir in parsley. Then drizzle over pork.

African Supper

INGREDIENTS

8 cups water

3 tsp. sea salt, divided

1 lb. dried lentils, rinsed, drained and picked over

1 cup + 2 Tbsp. extra-virgin olive oil

½ cup red wine vinegar

4 Tbsp. ground cumin, divided

2 Tbsp. + 2 ½ tsp. chili powder

1 tsp. garlic, minced

1 yellow onion, chopped

2 lbs. skinless, boneless chicken breast or turkey breast, thinly sliced

½ tsp. ground cinnamon

1 cup fresh parsley

Combine water and 1 tsp. salt in stock pot over high heat. Add lentils. Bring to a boil. Cover and reduce heat to medium. Simmer until lentils are soft, about 20 to 25 minutes. Drain well. Rinse under cold water and drain well. Place in large bowl and set aside.

In small bowl, mix 1 cup olive oil, vinegar, 2 Tbsp. cumin, 2 Tbsp. chili powder, garlic, and 1 tsp. sea salt. Pour this dressing over lentils. Toss gently and let cool.

In large skillet heat 2 tablespoons olive oil. Add onion and sauté until well cooked, about 5 minutes.

Onion should appear dark brown and soft. Add chicken or turkey and sauté 2 minutes more. Add 1 tsp. sea salt, 2 Tbsp. cumin, 2 ½ tsp. chili powder, and cinnamon. Sauté until poultry is cooked through.

Arrange lentils on a large serving platter. Place sliced chicken on top of lentils. Use remaining dressing and pour over chicken. Sprinkle with chopped parsley. Serve at room temperature.

SERVES

12

Lamb Chops

INGREDIENTS

2 tsp. ground cumin

1 tsp. ground coriander

1 tsp. ground cinnamon

½ tsp. freshly ground black pepper

1 ¼ lb. boneless lamb (top round), cut into strips

12 skewers, soaked in water for 20 minutes, if wooden

Preheat the grill or grill pan.

In a small bowl, combine the cumin, coriander, cinnamon, and pepper. In a large bowl, sprinkle the spice mixture over the lamb strips and toss to coat evenly.

Thread 1 piece of lamb onto each skewer and grill over medium-high heat for 4 to 5 minutes, turning once.

SERVES

4

Gyro Power

INGREDIENTS

½ cup white onion, cut into chunks

1 lb. ground lamb

1 lb. 96% ground lean ground beef

1 Tbsp. garlic, minced

1 ½ tsp. dried oregano

2 tsp. ground cumin

1 tsp. dried marjoram

1 tsp. ground dried rosemary

1 tsp. ground dried thyme

2 tsp. ground black pepper

½ tsp. parsley

Place the onion in a food processor, and process until finely chopped. Scoop the onions onto the center of a towel, gather up the ends of the towel, and squeeze out the liquid from the onions. Place the onions into a mixing bowl along with the lamb and beef. Season with the garlic, oregano, cumin, marjoram, rosemary, thyme, black pepper, and parsley. Mix well with your hands until well combined. Cover, and refrigerate 1 to 2 hours to allow the flavors to blend.

Preheat oven to 325 degrees.

Place the meat mixture into the food processor, and pulse for about a minute until finely chopped and the mixture feels tacky. Pack the meat mixture into a 7 x 4 inch loaf pan, making sure there are no air pockets. Line a roasting pan with a damp kitchen towel. Place the loaf pan on the towel, inside the roasting pan, and place into the preheated oven. Fill the roasting pan with boiling water to reach halfway up the sides of the loaf pan.

Bake until the gyro meat is no longer pink in the center, and the internal temperature registers 165 degrees on a meat thermometer, 45 minutes to 1 hour. Pour off any accumulated fat, and allow cooling slightly before slicing thinly and serving

Thai Curry Shrimp with Vegetables

INGREDIENTS

1 ½ Tbsp. extra-virgin olive oil

1 cup slivered carrots

1 yellow onion, chopped

1-13 oz. can light coconut milk

2 Tbsp. curry powder

1 red pepper

1 zucchini, halved lengthwise and sliced

1 cup sugar snap peas

16 oz. cooked shrimp, thawed and tailed removed

2 tsp. corn starch, dissolved in water

1 tsp. fish sauce

½ tsp. red pepper flakes (optional)

Heat olive oil in nonstick skillet. Add onions and peppers and cook for 3 minutes.

Add carrots and sugar snap peas and sauté for 3-5 minutes. Add zucchini and sauté an additional 2 minutes. Add shrimp, coconut milk, curry, fish sauce, and red pepper flakes. Keep over medium heat until warmed throughout.

SERVES

4

Mediterranean Shrimp

INGREDIENTS

1 Tbsp. extra-virgin olive oil

1 ½ cups green onion, diced

2 tsp. garlic, minced

2-14.5 oz. cans no-salt-added diced tomatoes, with their juices

¼ cup fresh parsley, finely minced

2 Tbsp. fresh dill, finely minced

1 ¼ lb. medium shrimp, peeled and deveined

¼ teaspoon freshly ground black pepper, plus more to taste

2/3 cup crumbled fat-free feta cheese

Preheat the oven to 425 degrees.

Heat the oil in an ovenproof skillet over medium-high heat. Add the onion and cook, stirring, until softened, about 3 minutes, then add the garlic and cook for 1 minute. Add the tomatoes and bring to a boil. Reduce the heat to medium-low and let simmer for about 5 minutes, until the tomato juices thicken.

Remove from the heat. Stir in the parsley, dill, and shrimp and season with pepper. Sprinkle the feta over the top. Bake until the shrimp are cooked though and the cheese melts, about 12 minutes.

SERVES

4

Kung Fu Shrimp

INGREDIENTS

1 Tbsp. Shaoxing (Chinese rice wine), dry sherry, or sake

1 tsp. cornstarch

1 lb. medium-size shrimp, peeled and deveined

Sauce Ingredients:

1 Tbsp. Stevia

2 Tbsp. water

1 Tbsp. Chinese black vinegar or balsamic vinegar

2 Tbsp. Braggs Amino Acid or tamari sauce

¾ tsp. cornstarch

½ tsp. dark sesame oil

Remaining Ingredients:

2 Tbsp. extra-virgin olive oil

1 1/3 cups green bell pepper, strips

2 Tbsp. garlic, minced

1 ½ Tbsp. ginger, peeled and minced

3 to 4 small dried hot red chilies, broken in half and seeded

¼ cup unsalted dry roasted peanuts, chopped

3 cups cooked brown rice

To prepare shrimp, combine first 3 ingredients; cover and chill 10 minutes.

To prepare sauce, combine sweetener and next 5 ingredients (through sesame oil).

Heat a 14-inch wok over high heat. Add olive oil to wok, swirling to coat. Add bell pepper, garlic, ginger, and chilies to wok; stir-fry 1 minute or just until chilies begin to lightly brown. Add shrimp mixture to wok, stir-fry 2 minutes or until shrimp are done. Stir sauce; add sauce to wok.

Stir-fry 30 seconds or until sauce thickens. Sprinkle with chopped peanuts. Serve over rice.

SERVES

4

Shrimp Scampi Sizzler

INGREDIENTS

2 Tbsp. extra-virgin olive oil

4 tsp. garlic, minced

1/3 cup shallots, finely sliced

1 ¼ lbs. large shrimp, peeled and deveined

1-14oz. can artichoke hearts, rinsed, drained, and quartered

1/3 cup dry white wine

2 Tbsp. fresh lemon juice

1 Tbsp. fresh lime juice

2 Tbsp. chopped fresh flat-leaf parsley, plus more for garnish

Ground black pepper, to taste

Heat the oil in a large skillet over medium heat. Add the garlic and shallots and cook, stirring, until softened but not browned, 2 to 3 minutes.

Add the shrimp, artichoke hearts, wine, lemon and lime juice and cook until the shrimp are cooked through, 3 to 4 minutes. Stir in parsley and pepper. Divide among 4 plates, garnish with additional parsley, and serve.

SERVES

4

Thai Coconut Curry Shrimp with Peppers

INGREDIENTS

1 tsp. extra-virgin olive oil

½ cup onion, chopped

1 yellow pepper, sliced in long strips

½ tsp. red curry paste (such as Thai kitchen)

1 tsp. Stevia

12 oz. large shrimp, peeled and deveined

1/3 cup light coconut milk

2 tsp. low sodium fish sauce

¼ cup green onions, chopped

Heat oil in a large nonstick skillet over medium-high heat. Add onion and curry paste to pan, and sauté 1 minute, stirring occasionally. Stir in sugar; sauté 15 seconds. Add shrimp; sauté 3 minutes or until shrimp are done, stirring frequently. Stir in coconut milk and fish sauce; cook 30 seconds or until thoroughly heated. Remove from heat; stir in green onions and yellow pepper slices.

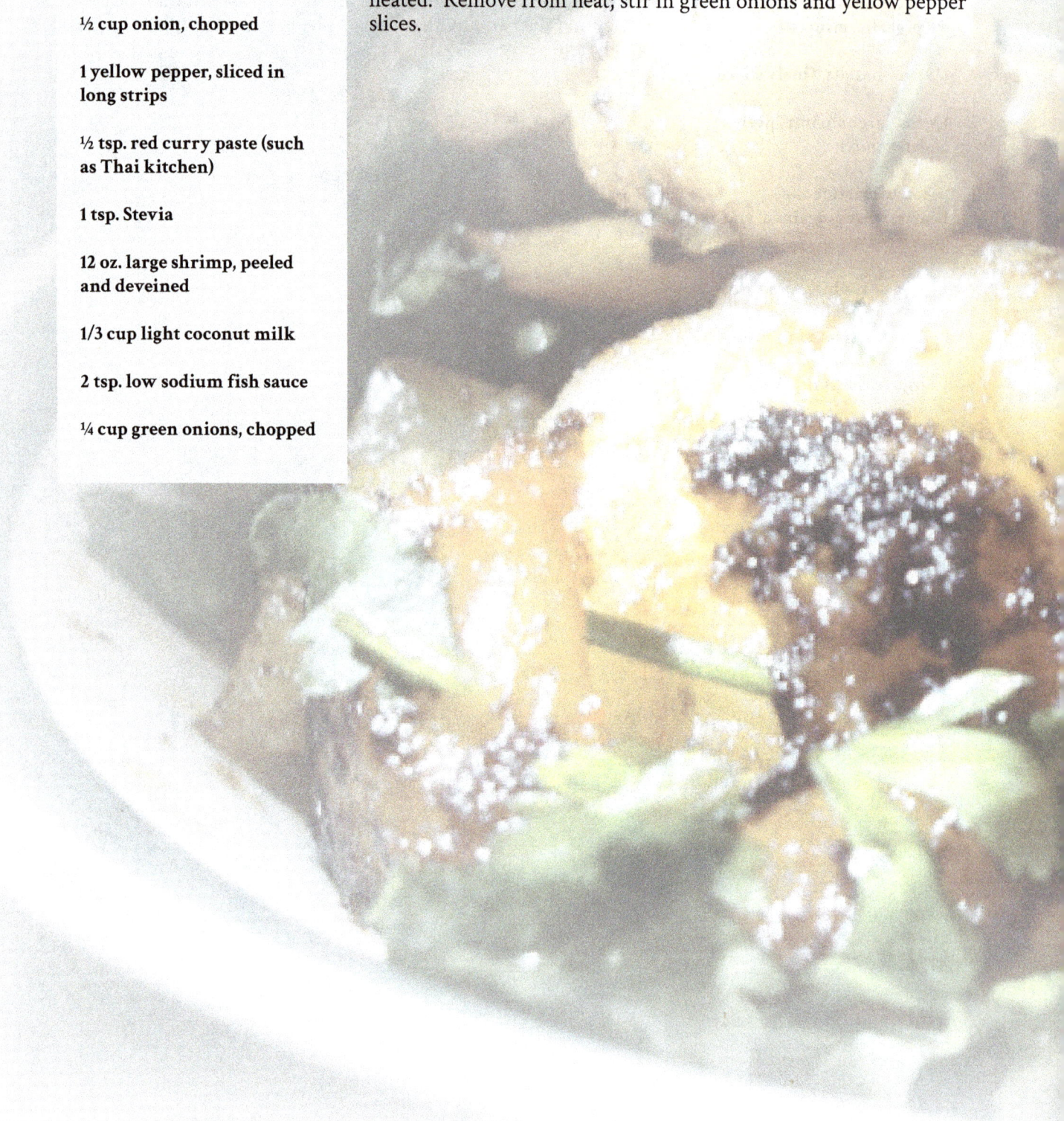

Healthy Creole

INGREDIENTS

1 celery rib, chopped

1 yellow onion, chopped

1 green pepper, chopped

1 Tbsp. extra-virgin olive oil

1-14.5 oz. can no salt added, diced tomatoes, do not drain

2 Tbsp. savory herb with garlic soup mix

½ tsp. garlic, minced

1 tsp. low sodium Worcestershire sauce

2 bay leaves

½ tsp. cayenne pepper

½ tsp. red pepper flakes

1 lb. cooked medium shrimp, peeled and deveined

2 cups cooked brown rice

In a large skillet, sauté the celery, onion, and green pepper in oil until tender. Add the tomatoes, soup mix, garlic, Worcestershire sauce, bay leaves, cayenne, and red pepper flakes. Bring to a boil. Reduce heat; cover and simmer for 15 minutes.

Add shrimp; heat through. Discard bay leaf. Serve with rice.

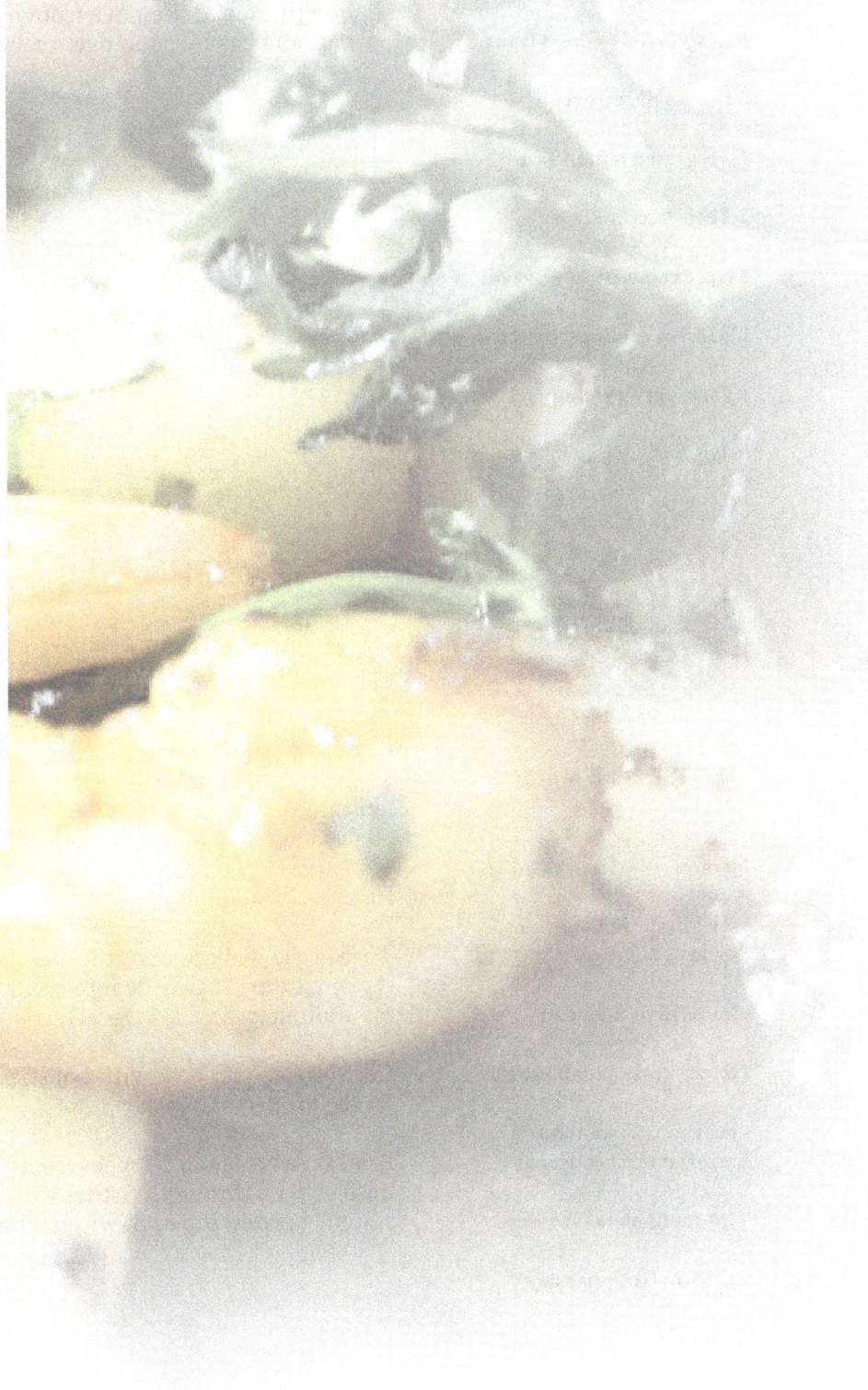

Dinner Scallops

INGREDIENTS

1 cup low-sodium chicken broth

1 ½ Tbsp. capers

1 ½ tsp. whole wheat flour

2 tsp. garlic, minced

1 tsp. grated lemon zest

2 Tbsp. lemon juice

3 tsp. extra-virgin olive oil

1 ½ lb. sea scallops, patted dry

1 Tbsp. parsley, chopped

½ tsp. basil

In a 2-cup liquid measure, stir broth, capers, flour, garlic, zest, and juice, until flour dissolves.

Heat 2 tsp. oil in large nonstick skillet over medium-high heat. Next add scallops and cook, turning once, 4 to 5 minutes until golden and cooked through. Remove to a plate.

Add broth mixture to skillet; bring to a boil; boil 1 minute until slightly thickened. Remove from heat; stir in remaining oil, parsley, and basil. Spoon over scallops.

SERVES 4

Sweet Scallops

INGREDIENTS

1 lemon

¼ cup organic honey or Stevia

¼ cup Dijon mustard

1 lb. sea scallops (about 20)

1 package (5.7 ounces) herb-flavored couscous

4 (10-inch) metal skewers

Garnish: fresh parsley

Grate rind from lemon to make 1 tsp. Squeeze lemon to make 1 Tbsp. lemon juice. Stir together lemon juice, honey/Stevia, and mustard in a bowl. Add scallops; toss to coat. Cover; refrigerate for 20 minutes.

Heat the broiler.

Thread the scallops onto the metal skewers, dividing equally. Pour the remaining marinade into a small saucepan; boil the marinade for 3 minutes.

Coat broiler-pan rack with nonstick cooking spray. Place skewers on the broiler-pan rack.

Broil skewers about 3 inches from heat for 4 minutes per side or until cooked through, basting with marinade. Divide couscous among 4 plates; top each with scallops and garnish with parsley.

SERVES 4

Salmon Patties

INGREDIENTS

1 lb. skinless salmon fillet, cut into 1-inch cubes

1 Tbsp. Dijon mustard

½ tsp. garlic, minced

1 Tbsp. grated lime peel

1 Tbsp. ginger, peeled and minced

1 Tbsp. fresh cilantro, chopped

1 tsp. Braggs Amino Acid or tamari sauce

1 tsp. ground coriander

Preheat the barbeque grill to medium-high heat. Coat grill rack with olive oil cooking spray

In a food processor, pulse the salmon just enough to grind it coarsely. Put that in a bowl and mix in mustard, garlic, lime peel, ginger, cilantro, Braggs Amino Acid/tamari sauce, and coriander.

Form into patties and season with Mrs. Dash seasonings.

Grill or cook in skillet—turning once until done (about 4 minutes per side for medium)

Salmon Surprise

INGREDIENTS

4-6 oz. salmon fillets, skinned

1 ½ tsp. ground coriander

Olive oil cooking spray

2 Tbsp. honey or Stevia

1 Tbsp. fresh lime juice

2 ½ tsp. Braggs Amino Acid or tamari sauce

1 teaspoon Sriracha

2 Tbsp. green onions, sliced

Sprinkle fish evenly with coriander. Heat a large nonstick skillet over medium-high heat. Coat pan with cooking spray. Add fish to pan; cook 4 minutes on each side or until fish flakes easily when tested with a fork or until desired degree of doneness.

Combine honey, juice, Braggs or tamari sauce, and Sriracha; drizzle over fish. Sprinkle with green onions.

Balsamic Salmon

INGREDIENTS

1 Tbsp. extra-virgin olive oil

4 wild-caught salmon fillets

1 tsp. cracked black pepper

1/3 cup balsamic vinegar

1 Tbsp. Stevia or organic honey

Heat oil in a large skillet over medium-high heat. Season both sides of salmon with cracked pepper. Add salmon to skillet and cook 1 to 2 minutes per side, until golden brown.

Meanwhile, in a small bowl, whisk together vinegar and Stevia/honey. Add vinegar mixture to skillet and simmer until fish is fork-tender and liquid reduces and thickens, about 2 minutes. For a thicker, reduced sauce, simmer for 3 to 5 additional minutes.

Serve with brown rice or rice pilaf.

SERVES

4

Pesto Baked Fish

INGREDIENTS

4 sheets parchment paper

4-6 oz. halibut, tilapia fillet, or any fish

4 Tbsp. store bought or homemade pesto sauce dressing section

1 cup carrots, shredded

1 cup zucchini, shredded

1 cup cabbage, shredded

2 tsp. garlic, minced

1 tsp. freshly ground pepper, divided

4 tsp. extra-virgin olive oil

4 tsp. low-sodium chicken stock

Olive oil cooking spray

Preheat oven to 450 degrees. Unfold parchment and coat lightly with cooking spray. Leave one two- inch edge ungreased. Place fillet on one side so it touches the fold but not the ungreased edge. Spread 1 Tbsp. pesto over fillet and top with ¼ cup each, carrot, cabbage, and zucchini. Sprinkle with pepper and garlic. Drizzle fillet with 1 tsp. oil and 1 tsp. chicken stock. Fold paper and seal edges with narrow folds.

Repeat with the remaining parchment paper, fish, and vegetables. Place packets on baking sheets, and bake for 15 minutes or until puffy and lightly browned. To serve, open packets and transfer the fillet with their vegetable topping to plates. Pour juices over top. Or serve right in packets.

SERVES

4

Sweet Tuna Salad

INGREDIENTS

1 can tuna, drained

2 Tbsp. plain Greek yogurt

1 Tbsp. honey mustard

5-7 cherry tomatoes, halved

5-7 red or green grapes, halved

Combine all ingredients and mix well.

Can be mixed with lettuce or spinach

Shrimp Lettuce Wraps

INGREDIENTS

4 oz. shrimp (pre-cooked and frozen)

¼ cup avocado, cubed

1/8 cup carrots, grated

1/8 cup cucumber, grated

1/8 cup edamame beans

1/8 cup navy beans (cooked or canned), drained

1 Tbsp. Asian Dressing

1/8 cup fat-free plain yogurt

3 iceberg lettuce leaves

Combine defrosted shrimp, avocado, carrots, and cucumber together in a mixing bowl. Gently mix in beans, dressing, and yogurt.

Lay lettuce leaves on countertop. Divide mixture evenly among leaves. (Depending on the size of your leaves, you may need more or less.) You can also choose to serve the remaining mixture as a side salad with the wraps.

Roll it up like a tortilla shell. Fold the bottom up, fold in the two sides, and roll.

Thai-Chicken Lettuce Wraps

INGREDIENTS

2 Tbsp. hoisin sauce

1 Tbsp. of Natural Peanut Butter

2 Tbsp. Braggs Amino Acid

2 ½ tsp. hot-pepper sauce

2 Tbsp. minced garlic

1 cup onion, minced

½ lb. ground chicken breast

2 tsp. fresh ginger, minced

1 tsp. toasted sesame oil

8 small leaves butter lettuce

1 whole green onion, chopped

1 small cucumber, seeded and sliced into 1-inch strips

In a medium bowl, combine the bamboo shoots, water chestnuts, sherry, hoisin sauce, peanut butter, Braggs, hot-pepper sauce, and Stevia. Mix well. Set aside.

Mist a large, nonstick skillet with olive oil spray and set over medium heat. Add the garlic and cook for 2 minutes, or until fragrant. Add the onion. Cook, stirring occasionally, for 3-4 minutes, or until tender and just starting to brown. Increase the heat to medium-high. Add the chicken and ginger. Cook, breaking the chicken into small chunks, for 3-4 minutes, or until no longer pink. Add the reserved bamboo shoot mixture. Cook for 2 minutes, or until hot. Stir in the sesame oil. Remove the pan from the heat. Spoon the chicken mixture, evenly divided, into the lettuce leaves. Set on a serving dish. Top with green onion and cucumber. Serve immediately.

Chicken Taco Pita or Wrap

INGREDIENTS

2 ½ cup boneless, skinless cooked chicken, diced

¼ cup salsa

½ cup peppers, chopped

1/3 cup green onions, chopped

1 cup fat-free plain Greek yogurt

1 tsp. cumin

1/3 cup cilantro or parsley, chopped

Combine all ingredients and divide into 3 pitas. Cut in half or 3-4 large tortilla wraps. Top with lettuce, olives, and tomatoes.

SERVES

6

Tandoori Chicken Pitas

INGREDIENTS

¼ cup whole wheat flour

2 ½ Tbsp. curry powder

4 boneless, skinless chicken breast halves

1 Tbsp. extra-virgin olive oil

Yogurt Sauce Ingredients:

¾ cup fat-free Greek yogurt

2 Tbsp. red onion, finely chopped

2 tsp. garlic, minced

½ tsp. each ground cumin and salt

1 yellow bell pepper

2 cucumbers

4 whole wheat pitas

Garnish: lime wedges and chopped cilantro

Mix flour, curry powder, and pepper in a plastic food bag. Add chicken, close bag and shake to coat.

Remove chicken; shake off excess flour.

Meanwhile, heat oil in a large nonstick skillet over medium-high heat. Add chicken and cook, turning once, 10 minutes or until golden and cooked through. Remove to a cutting board.

While chicken cooks, mix sauce ingredients in a bowl. Coarsely chop bell pepper, tomatoes, and cucumbers; toast pitas.

Cut chicken diagonally into wide strips. Place a pita on each plate. Top with pepper, tomato, and cucumber then chicken. Spoon on sauce; garnish with limes and cilantro.

SERVES

4

Focus on how you **feel** after eating something. Listening to your own body is one of your greatest tools in achieving and maintaining optimal health!

Avocado Tuna Pita Panini

INGREDIENTS

1 avocado, peeled and pitted

1 clove garlic, minced

1 lemon, juiced

1-2 pouches tuna in water

Whole-wheat pitas, halved

4 oz alfalfa sprouts

1 cucumber, thinly sliced

Handful of cherry tomatoes, halved

In a medium bowl, combine avocado, garlic, and lemon juice and mix well with a fork.

Divide tuna, sprouts, cucumber, and tomato evenly into pita halves.

Toast pita in toaster oven, on the stove, or on a griddle until the outside is crispy and lightly browned. Top with avocado spread before serving.

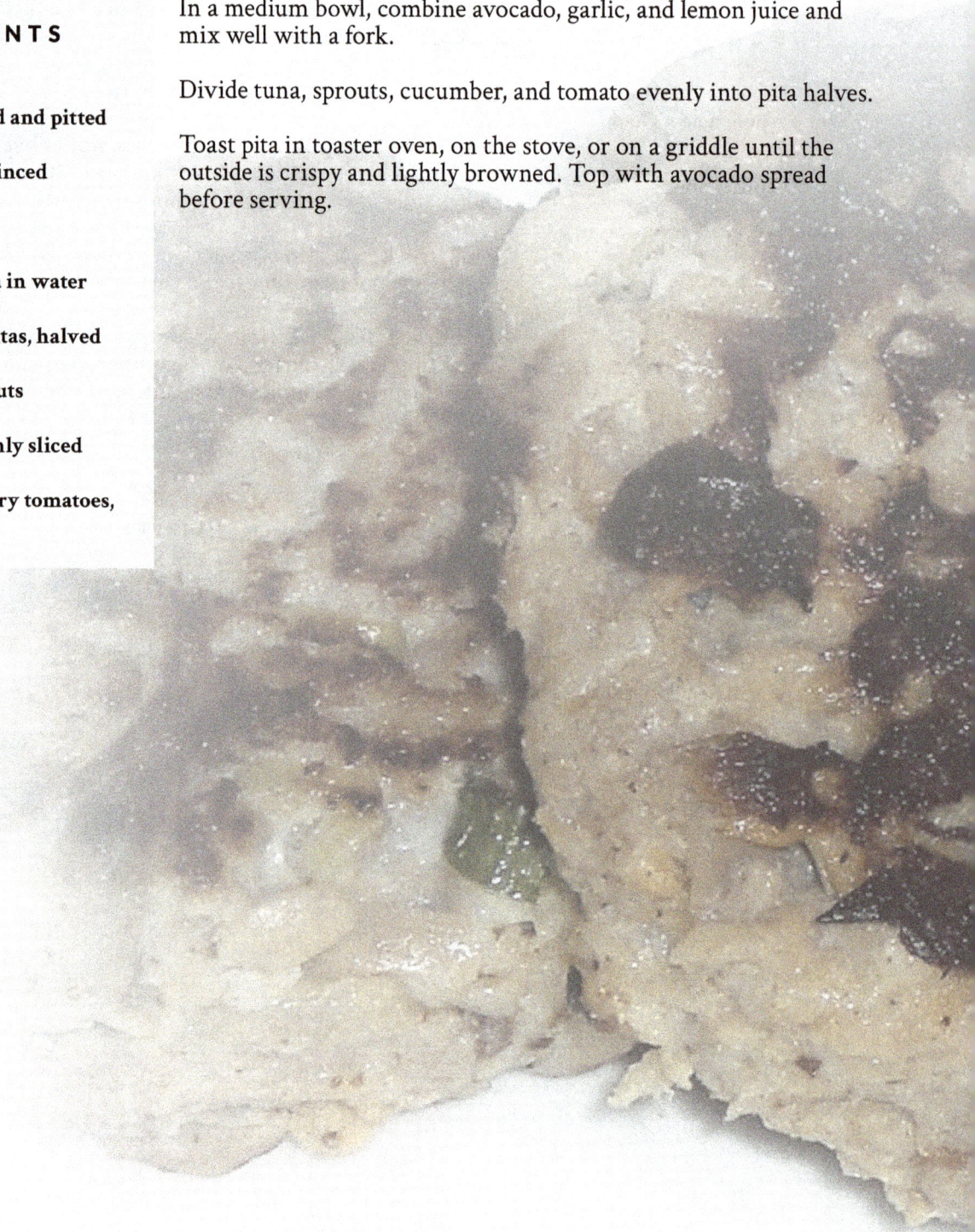

Fast Tuna Burgers

INGREDIENTS

2 lb. fresh tuna steak

3 tsp. garlic, minced

2 Tbsp. Braggs Amino Acid or
tamari sauce

2 Tbsp. unsulfured molasses

3 green onions, finely
chopped

½ sweet red pepper, finely
chopped

½ Vidalia onion, finely
chopped

2 tsp. sesame oil

1 Tbsp. Mrs. Dash seasoning
of your choice

Olive oil cooking spray

4 Ezekiel grain buns or 100%
whole wheat sandwich thins

2 tsp. fresh dill

Place tuna in food processor and pulse until meat resembles texture of ground turkey or beef. In large mixing bowl combine garlic, Braggs or tamari sauce, molasses, green onions, red pepper, Vidalia onions, sesame oil, herbal seasoning, and dill. Add tuna. With clean bare hands, mix all ingredients until uniformly distributed. Divide into four parts and shape into flat patties.

Coat grill pan with olive oil spray. Place over medium heat. Place patties in grill pan, cook for 2 minutes and flip. Cook for another 2 minutes. This will make a rare burger. If you want your burger medium to well done, cook for another 2 minutes on both sides.

Meanwhile, spread bottom half of you bun with hummus. Place lettuce greens of your choice on top and set the burger on top of that. Add condiments of your choice and serve immediately.

SERVES

4

Chicken & Mushroom Crepes

INGREDIENTS

1 large egg

2 large egg whites

¾ cup whole wheat pastry flour

1 cup almond or rice milk

Olive oil cooking spray

1 cup onions, chopped

½ cup white mushrooms, sliced

2 cups boneless, skinless chicken breast, chopped

2 Tbsp. dry white wine

4 cups baby spinach

1 tsp. dried tarragon

3 oz. soft goat cheesed

1 oz. low-fat, low sodium shredded Swiss cheese

2 tsp. basil leaves

2 medium Roma tomatoes, chopped

Prepare crepes: In a blender, combine egg and egg whites, flour, and milk. Process until well mixed, scraping down sides of blender jar to incorporate flour well. Chill blender jar full of batter in refrigerator for 1 hour. Remove blender jar and put lack on base; pulse to re-mix batter. Heat an 8- inch nonstick crepe pan or small sauté pan over medium-high heat. When hot, mist with cooking spray. Add ¼ cup batter, then swirl to coat pan. Cook until crepe is set, about 1 minute. Run a spatula around edges and flip, cooking for just a few seconds after flipping. Invert pan over a cutting board to drop crepe onto the board and allow crepe to cook. Repeat until you have 8 crepes.

Mist a cast-iron or nonstick skillet with cooking spray and sauté onions over medium heat. When onions start to soften and brown, about 5 minutes, add mushrooms and chicken and stir. Over medium-high heat, sear chicken undisturbed for a few minutes to allow it to brown nicely. Once browned, stir occasionally until chicken is cooked through and mushrooms are tender, about 5 minutes. Add wine and cook, stirring, until wine reduces by half. Add spinach, tarragon, and basil, and stir, turning leaves until they are wilted and bright green. Move contents of pan to 1 side and add cheese to the other side. Mash cheese with your spatula to melt, then stir into chicken mixture. Remove skillet from heat and allow mixture to cool slightly.

Preheat oven to 375 degrees. Assemble crepes: Measure ¼ cup portions of chicken mixture into the center of each crepe, then roll up and place on a baking pan or casserole. Top with Swiss cheese,dividing evenly, and bake for 20 minutes. Garnish with tomatoes and serve.

SERVES

4

Cocoa Chicken Mole

INGREDIENTS

2 Tbsp. extra-virgin olive oil

1 yellow onion, chopped

1 ½ tsp. garlic, minced

1 chipotle pepper + 1 tsp. adobo sauce from can, chopped

1 cup no sugar added raisins

2 cups canned no salt added tomatoes, chopped

3 Tbsp. smooth natural peanut butter

2 cups low-sodium chicken broth

2 ½ tsp. chili powder

1 tsp. ground cinnamon

1 ½ oz. unsweetened chocolate or 2 Tbsp. unsweetened cocoa powder

1 rotisserie chicken, meat removed and shredded

Fresh cilantro, for serving

Lime wedges, for serving

1 avocado, sliced, for serving

100% whole wheat tortilla

Place a pot over medium heat and coat with the oil. Add the onion and garlic, stirring to soften for 5 minutes. Add the chipotle with adobo sauce, raisins, and tomatoes, stirring to combine. Bring to a simmer and cook for 10 minutes.

Carefully pour the mixture into a blender. Add the peanut butter, broth, chili powder, and cinnamon. Puree the mixture until smooth.

Return the mixture to the pot over medium heat. Cook for 15 minutes, stirring occasionally. Add the chocolate and stir until melted. Add the shredded chicken and heat through.

Serve with cilantro, lime, avocado, and tortillas.

SERVES

5

Green Chicken Salad

INGREDIENTS

3 cups cooked (organic) chicken, diced

1 medium-ripe avocado; pitted, peeled and mashed

1 stalk celery, chopped

1 green pepper, chopped

½ small onion

2 Tbsp. Greek Yogurt

1 Tbsp. mustard

Ground black pepper to taste

Combine all ingredients and mix well.

Can serve on 100% Whole Wheat bread/tortilla, or a lettuce wrap.

Sweet Chicken Salad

INGREDIENTS

2-3 cooked chicken breasts (organic), shredded

½ cup red onion, chopped

½ cup red apple, peeled and diced

2/3 cup green grapes, halved

¼ cup Greek yogurt

1 lemon

½ tsp garlic powder

Ground black pepper to taste

In a large bowl, combine all ingredients. Add ground pepper to taste. Eat plain, wrap in lettuce, on 100%

Whole Wheat bread/tortilla, or mix with spinach/lettuce to create a salad.

Healthy Fish Wraps

INGREDIENTS

Ingredients for Bubble Bee Salad:

1 cup dried black beans

1 cup red onion, chopped

3 small jalapeno pepper, seeded and chopped

Juice of 1 lime

2/3 packed cup fresh cilantro, chopped

2 tsp. chili powder, divided

1 ½ Tbsp. Olive oil for coating grill or olive oil cooking spray for skillet

Fresh ground black pepper, to taste

½ cup cilantro

Ingredients:

1 Bubble Bee Salad

2 (6 oz. each) grilled tilapia fillets, or other fish, cut into bite-size pieces

Olive oil cooking spray

4 whole-wheat tortillas (8 inches each)

1 small Roma tomato, seeded and chopped

1 cup spinach leaves, roughly chopped

In a blender or food processor fitted with a metal blade, puree Bubble Bee Salad to a spreadable, slightly chunky paste. Microwave tilapia for about 30 seconds to reheat.

Coat a medium skillet with cooking spray and set over medium heat. Warm tortillas in skillet 1 at a time, about 30 second per side. Alternatively, heat tortillas in microwave for 12 seconds each.

Place each tortilla on a plate. Spread about 3 Tbsp. Bubble Bee Salad mixture down the center of each tortilla. Top salad mixture with quarter of tilapia, quarter of tomato, and quarter of spinach. Tightly roll up tortillas to enclose filling. Cut each wrap in half on the diagonal and serve.

101
SERVES

Tuna Wrap

INGREDIENTS

½ cup canned tuna, drained

¼ cup fat-free cottage cheese

1 Tbsp. low-fat Italian dressing

1 tsp. sun-dried tomato, chopped

¼ cup yellow pepper, diced

1 tsp. garlic, chopped

2 tsp. dried basil

2 whole romaine lettuce leaves

In a bowl, combine tuna, cottage cheese, dressing, tomato, pepper, garlic, and basil. Mix well. Place all ingredients on top of lettuce leaf. Fold edges over and wrap.

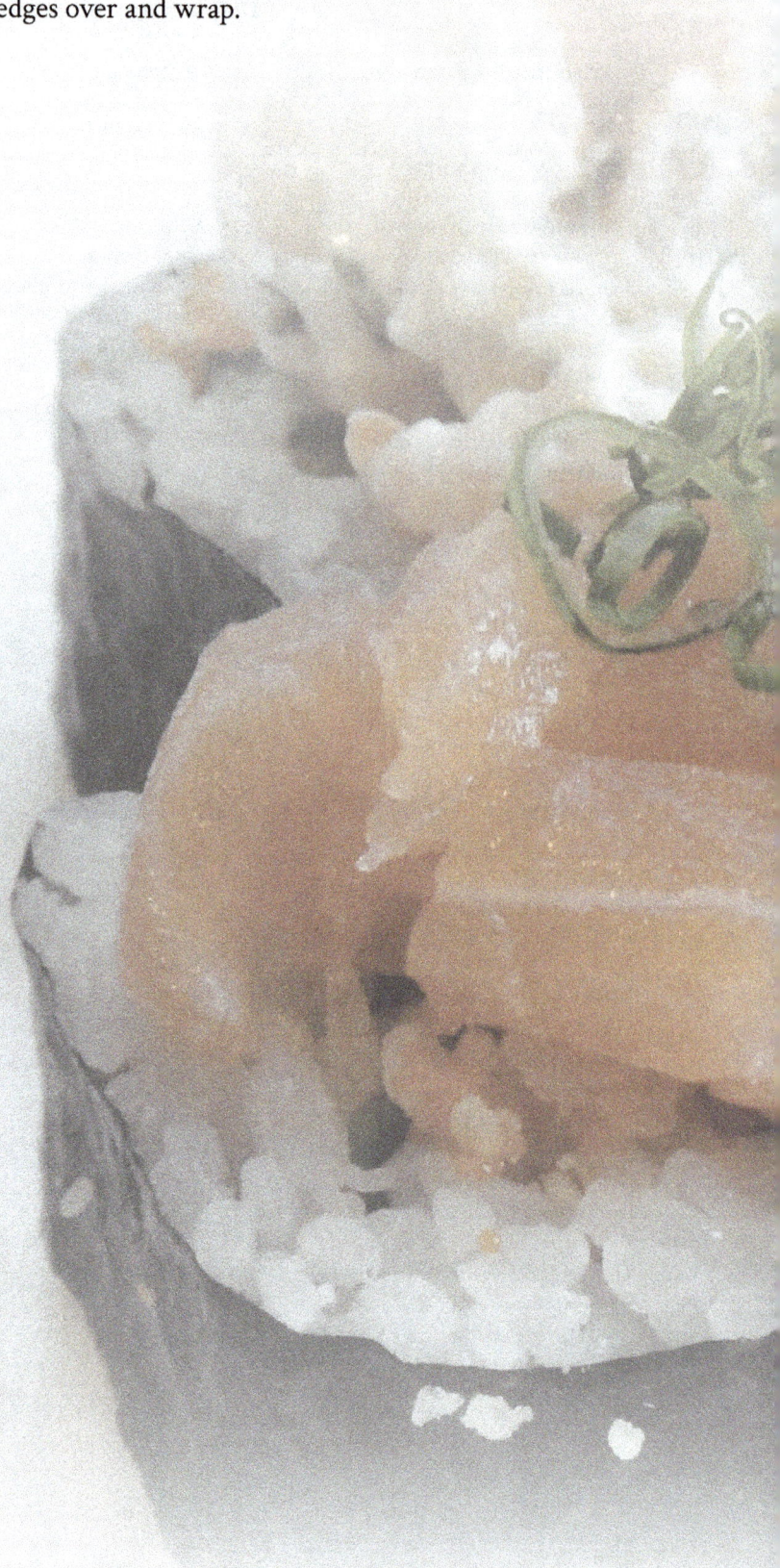

Healthy "Sushi" Wrap

INGREDIENTS

1 Tbsp. rice vinegar

2 tsp. fresh ginger, fined chopped

3 Tbsp. red onion, thinly shaved

¼ cup fat-free Greek yogurt

1 ½ tsp. wasabi paste

2 whole wheat tortillas

¼ small avocado, pitted and thinly sliced

½ cup carrot sticks, thinly sliced

1 cup cucumber, seeded and thinly sliced

1 ½ cup baby spinach, chopped

4 large shrimp, cooked, peeled, deveined, and chopped

In a small bowl, whisk together honey and vinegar (if honey does not dissolve, microwave for about 45 seconds). Add ginger and onion and toss to coat. Let stand for at least 20 minutes.

In another small bowl, stir together yogurt and wasabi.

On each tortilla, pile half of each of the following: avocado, carrots, cucumber, and spinach. Then top with shrimp and ginger mixture, dividing evenly. Drizzle each with yogurt sauce and roll up tortilla.

How to pack your "sushi" wrap for lunch:

Place a 12-inch piece of wax or parchment paper on your counter in a diamond position. Place filled tortilla in the center. Fold bottom edge of paper toward the center.

Fold right edge of paper across the wrap.

Fold left edge of paper over and continue to roll it around the wrap completely.

Twist top of paper, enclosing wrap, but be careful not to crush tortilla or filling. When you're ready to eat, simply untwist and tear away top end and use the paper to keep the wrap rolled together.

Elegant Egg White Sandwich

INGREDIENTS

4 large Eggland's Best eggs

½ tsp. ground turmeric

½ cup cauliflower, broken into very small florets

2 Tbsp. carrot, shredded

2 Tbsp. sliced water chestnuts, chopped

3 unsweetened dried apricots, chopped

2 Tbsp. fat-free Greek yogurt

1 tsp. lemon zest

1 ½ fresh lemon juice

1 ½ tsp. fresh ginger, chopped

1 tsp. curry powder

3 Tbsp. fresh cilantro leaves, chopped

4 slices multigrain bread, toasted

4 lettuce leaves

Place eggs in a 2-qt saucepan and cover with cold water. Place on stove over high heat and bring to a rolling boil. As soon as eggs start to boil, cover and remove from heat. Let stand for 15 minutes, then drain and rinse with cold water. Chill eggs in refrigerator or in a bowl of ice water until cook enough to handle, about 10 minutes.

In a 1-qt pot, bring 2 cups water to a boil and add turmeric. Add cauliflower and boil for 3 minutes, then drain and chill until ready to use.

Peel eggs and remove whites. Coarsely mash whites in a large bowl. Add cauliflower, carrot, water chestnuts, and apricots. In a small bowl, stir together yogurt, lemon zest and juice, honey, ginger, curry powder, and cilantro. Pour yogurt mixture over egg mixture and stir to combine.

Divide egg salad into 2 portions and spread onto 2 slices of bread, then add lettuce and top with remaining slices of bread.

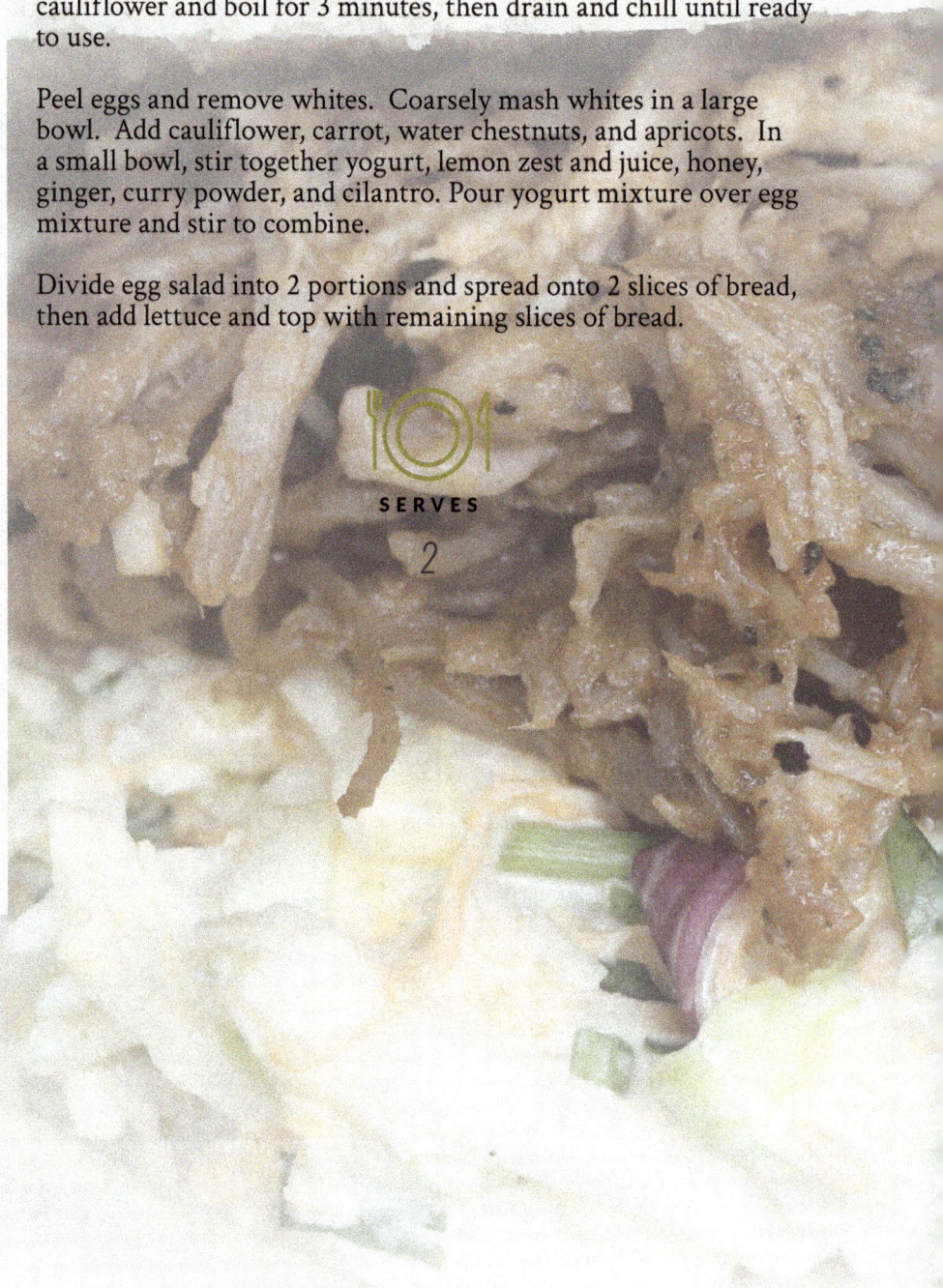

SERVES

2

BBQ Sandwich

INGREDIENTS

1 Tbsp. whole wheat flour

¼ tsp. garlic powder

1/8 tsp. onion powder

1 lb. top round roast or steak, extra-lean, cut into ¾-inch cubes

Olive oil cooking spray

¾ cup low-fat, low-sodium beef broth

2 Tbsp. Frank's Hot Buffalo sauce

1/3 cup barbecue sauce

1 cup white onion strips

4-100% whole wheat sandwich thins

In a medium plastic bag, combine flour, garlic powder, and onion powder. Add beef and shake bag until beef is evenly coated. Refrigerate beef for at least 15 minutes.

Preheat a medium, nonstick saucepan over medium-high heat. When it's hot, lightly mist pan with spray, then add beef. Brown beef on all sides, about 1 minute per side, then reduce heat to medium. Add broth and Frank's Hot Buffalo sauce. When liquid comes to a boil, reduce heat to low (liquid should still be boiling slightly). Cover and cook beef, stirring occasionally, for 1 to 1 ½ hours or until it's very tender. (The pieces should easily fall apart when smashed with a fork.) Using a slotted spoon, drain any excess liquid from beef and transfer the liquid to a medium bowl. Using a fork, separate pieces so beef is somewhat shredded, then mix in barbecue sauce.

During the last 5 minutes of cooking the beef, lightly mist a small, nonstick frying pan with spray and place it over medium heat. Add onion strips and cook until tender, about 5 minutes.

Meanwhile, place bun halves, inside down, in a medium, nonstick frying pan over medium heat. Cook until just toasted, about 2 to 4 minutes. Place each bun bottom on a plate. Pile ¼ of beef mixture onto each bun. Top with ¼ of onion strips. Add bun tops. Serve immediately.

SERVES

4

Mediterranean Burgers

INGREDIENTS

8 Portobello mushrooms, stemmed and cleaned

1 Tbsp. extra-virgin olive oil

20 oz. extra lean ground turkey

3 tsp. fresh thyme, chopped

1 tsp. garlic, minced

½ red onion, chopped

1 red bell pepper, chopped

1 large tomato, chopped

1 ½ Tbsp. red wine vinegar

½ cup fat-free plain yogurt

1 tsp. extra fine capers, drained

4 cornichons, chopped fine

2 Tbsp. fresh parsley, chopped rough

Preheat a grill or grill pan on medium-high heat.

Rub the portabellas lightly with the olive oil and season with black pepper.

Place on the grill and cook for 3 to 4 minutes on each side or until tender and cooked through.

Remove the mushrooms from the grill to a plate lined with paper towels to catch any excess moisture.

In a large mixing bowl combine the turkey, thyme, and garlic and mix well to combine.

Portion the turkey into four 5 oz. patties about ¾ inches thick.

Grill the turkey patties for about 4 to 5 minutes on each side or until a meat thermometer reads 165 degrees in the center of the patties.

Remove burgers from the grill and let rest for 4 minutes.

Mix the red onion, bell pepper, and tomato in a medium-mixing bowl.

Add the red wine vinegar and mix well, season with black pepper.

Ina separate mixing bowl, combine the yogurt, capers, cornichons, and parsley and mix well.

To serve, place a Portobello mushroom with the stem side up on a serving plate. Place the burger on top of the mushroom and top with the vegetable mixture followed by a spoonful of the yogurt sauce. Top with another Portobello, stem side down.

Repeat with the remaining four burgers, and serve immediately

Lean Turkey Burgers

INGREDIENTS

1 cup high-protein, 100% whole wheat cereal flakes

½ cup almond or rice milk

3 tsp. instant low-sodium chicken bouillon

3 Tbsp. yellow onion, minced

2 egg whites

2 Tbsp. fresh dill, sprigs pulled off the steams

1 lb. extra lean ground turkey

Combine first six ingredients in a large bowl. Let the milk soak into the cereal flakes for 5 minutes. Add extra lean ground turkey. Mix well with clean bare hands. Shape into patties and grill.

Serve hot with lightly toasted Ezekiel buns or 100% whole wheat sandwich thins. Avoid high-fat condiments such as mayonnaise. But can add mustard, low-sodium, low-sugar no high fructose corn syrup ketchup, lettuce, and slices of fresh tomato.

SERVES

6

Killer Sloppy Joes

INGREDIENTS

1 tsp. garlic, minced

1 small yellow onion

1 small green pepper

12 oz. lean ground turkey

¾ cup no high fructose corn syrup, no salt added ketchup

2 Tbsp. Worcestershire sauce

2/3 cup water

1 tsp. chili powder

Olive oil cooking spray

Chop all the vegetables roughly. Spray pan with cooking spray and cook veggies for about 4 minutes.

Add turkey with the vegetable mixture. When turkey is done cooking, add the ketchup, water, powders, Worcestershire sauce, and bring to a simmer. Heat buns for 1 minute and serve.

Shroom Focaccia

INGREDIENTS

1 Tbsp. extra-virgin olive oil

6 oz. mushrooms, sliced

1 whole-wheat focaccia bread (10-12 inch)

¾ cup fat-free mozzarella cheese, shredded

1 can (14.5 oz) no-salt added diced tomatoes, drained

3 Tbsp. fresh basil leaves, chopped

Heat oven to 350 degrees. In 8-inch skillet, heat oil over medium heat. Cook mushrooms in oil 3-4 minutes, stirring frequently, until tender. Drain if necessary.

On ungreased cookie sheet, place bread. Sprinkle ½ cup of the cheese on bread. Top with mushrooms and tomatoes. Sprinkle with remaining ¼ cup cheese.

Bake 15-20 minutes or until cheese is melted and bread is hot. Sprinkle with basil.

Chicken & Mushroom Focaccia

INGREDIENTS

8 oz. boneless, skinless chicken breast

1 medium Portobello mushroom

1 ½ Tbsp. fresh rosemary

1 tsp. fresh thyme

1 tsp. extra-virgin olive oil

1 ½ tsp. balsamic vinegar

2-3oz. whole wheat focaccia (about 4x5 inches each)

½ cup fat-free mozzarella cheese, thinly sliced

1 large tomato, thinly sliced

2 small scallions, chopped

½ cup fresh basil, thinly sliced

Preheat oven to 400 degrees. Line a sheet pan with nonstick foil, if desired. Sliced chicken into ½- inch strips, across the grain, and placed in a large bowl. Slice mushroom in slightly thinner strips and add to chicken. Sprinkle with rosemary and thyme. In a small bowl, stir together oil and vinegar, then drizzle over chicken-mushroom mixture. Spread mixture out on prepared pan, not allowing strips to touch, and roast for 15 minutes, stirring halfway through. Remove from oven to cook slightly.

Slice focaccia horizontally, creating top and bottom halves, and toast in a toaster or under a hot broiler for 1 minute to crisp, if desired. To assemble, place toasted focaccia on plates. Place half of cheese on each bottom half, followed by half of chicken-mushroom mixture. Divide tomato, scallions, and basil between the 2 sandwiches and cover with top halves.

SERVES
2

Whole Wheat Pizza Dough

INGREDIENTS

1 Tbsp. raw organic honey, Stevia or agave nectar

1 cup less 1 ½ Tbsp. lukewarm water, divided

1 package active dry yeast

2 ½ cups 100% whole wheat flour, divided

4 tsp. vital wheat gluten

½ tsp. sea salt

Pinch of cinnamon

3 Tbsp. extra-virgin olive oil, divided

In a large bowl, mix together honey and 1/3 cup water. Sprinkle in yeast and allow to proof, undisturbed (do not stir or move bowl), for 10 minutes or until yeast is foamy. (NOTE: If yeast does not foam, it is dead and your dough will not rise. Discard and start again with fresh ingredients.)

While yeast is proofing, mix together 2 cups flour, wheat gluten, salt, and cinnamon in another large bowl. Once yeast is foamy, add remaining water and 2 Tbsp. oil to yeast mixture. Pour in flour mixture and gently fold in with a bowl scraper or spatula until just combined. Mixture will form a very wet ball. Coat the bottom of another large bowl with remaining oil (ensure that bowl is large enough so that, when doubled in size, the dough will not reach the top). Transfer dough to bowl, rolling ball a bit to coat with oil. Cover bowl tightly with plastic wrap and set aside at room temperature to rise for 1 hour. Dough will be very soft and sticky.

Lightly dust counter with about ¼ cup flour. Transfer dough to floured surface and roll lightly in flour, dusting your hands with additional remaining flour as needed. Gently knead dough, using remaining flour as needed, for about 1 minute. Form dough into a ball and place back into bowl. Cover bowl again tightly with plastic wrap and set aside at room temperature to rise for 30 minutes.

Transfer dough back to floured surface, adding more flour to prevent dough from sticking, if needed, and cut dough in half to form 2 balls. Lightly knead each for about 30 seconds and reform into balls.

Dough is now ready to be formed into pizza crust or wrapped for future use. To store, wrap each dough ball individually in plastic wrap. Dough can be kept refrigerated for 24 hours or frozen for up to 1 month.

To use from refrigerator just remove dough from fridge and allow warming a little at room temperature for about 10 minutes. Form a pizza crust. To use from frozen just transfer dough from freezer to fridge and allow to defrost over night before following directions "from refrigerator" steps above.

Serves: Makes 2, 1 lb. dough balls

To make this whole wheat pizza dough Gluten-Free:

Swap 100% whole wheat flour for an all-purpose gluten-free baking flour mix Remove vital wheat gluten from recipe Increase yeast to 2 packages

Add 1 tsp. baking powder to flour mixture Reduce water to 1/3 cup total

Add 1/3 cup egg whites in Step Three when adding flour to proofed yeast

Have a bit of extra water on hand in case mixture is dry

Add 4 tsp. xanthan gum to dry ingredients

Add 2 tsp. apple cider vinegar after combining yeast and dry ingredients

Pacific Pizza

INGREDIENTS

100% Whole Wheat prepared pizza crust Boboli (brand)

¾ cup low-fat, low-sodium marinara sauce

1 cup grape tomatoes, halved and broiled until softened

½ cup green onion, chopped

½ cup crumbled fat-free feta cheese

8 oz. medium shrimp, peeled and deveined

1 ½ Tbsp. fresh oregano, chopped

¼ cup black olives (optional)

Preheat oven at 450 degrees.

Spread ½ cup marinara sauce on pizza crust. Then top with grape tomatoes, halved and broiled until softened.

Add onions, feta cheese, shrimp, and black olives, then bake for 15 minutes or until shrimp are cooked through and crust is golden brown.

Sprinkle with chopped fresh oregano. Cut into 5 slices, and serve.

SERVES

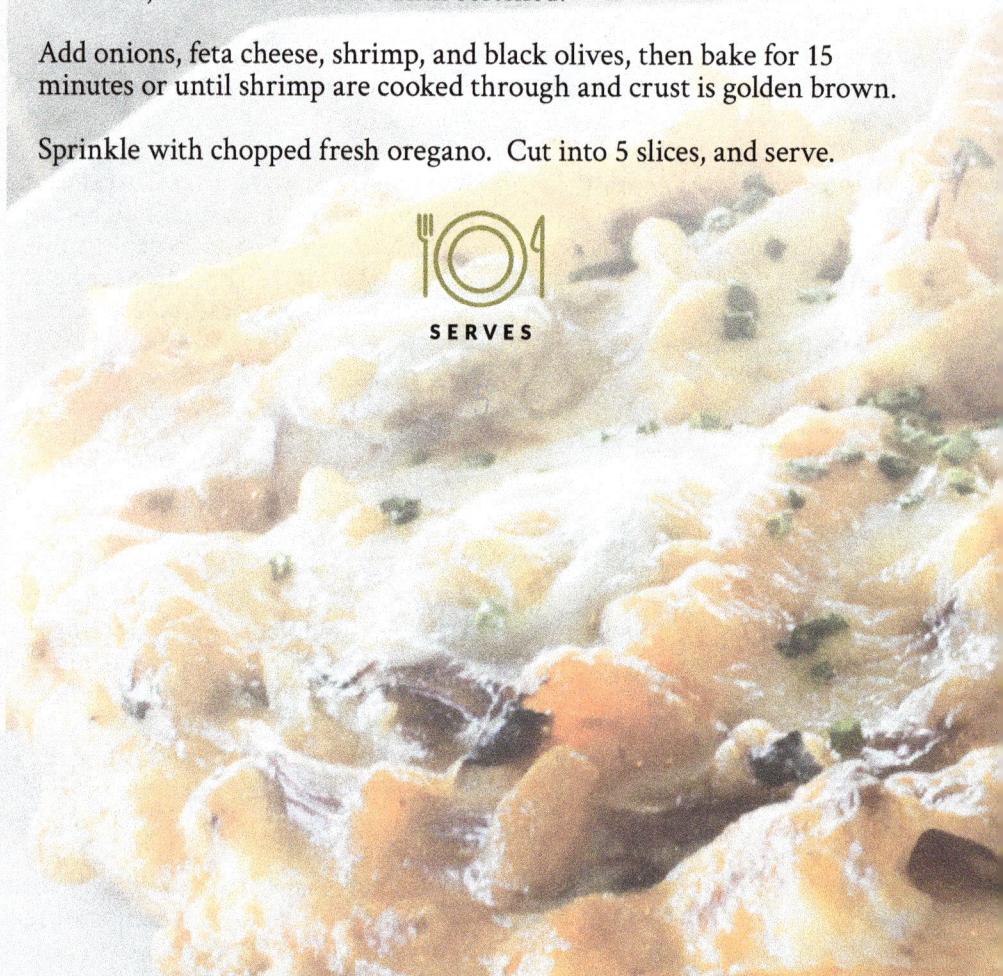

> Drink plenty of water. Many people go through life dehydrated which causes tiredness, low energy, and headaches. Water helps flush our systems of waste products and toxins and decreases water retention and inflammation.

Mediterranean Dream Pizza

INGREDIENTS

1 Tbsp. extra-virgin olive oil

1 Tbsp. garlic, minced

½ tsp. chili powder

½ red sweet bell pepper, cut in half

½ orange sweet bell pepper, cut in half

1 red onion, peeled and sliced into ½-inch thick rings

½ each medium green and yellow zucchini, sliced lengthwise

1-1 lb. ball Whole Wheat Pizza Dough or 1-1 lb. package store-bought whole wheat pizza dough

1/8 cup black olives

Olive oil cooking spray

Baba Ghanoush Ingredients:

1 large eggplant

½ cup flat-leaf parsley sprigs, coarsely chopped

•3 Tbsp. tahini (sesame seed paste)

3 Tbsp. fresh lemon juice

1 Tbsp. extra-virgin olive oil

2 tsp. garlic

½ tsp. cumin

Preheat grill to medium heat.

Pierce eggplant several times with a fork and place directly onto grill. Roast eggplant, turning occasionally, until skin is charred and eggplant is tender throughout when pierced with a knife, about 15 to 18 minutes.

Remove from grill and let cool at room temperature for about 10 minutes.

While eggplant is cooking, mix together oil, 1 Tbsp. water, minced garlic, and chili powder. Brush bell peppers, onion, zucchini, and olives with mixture. Grill peppers, onion, zucchini, and olives over medium heat until lightly charred and tender, about 6 to 8 minutes. Let cool slightly at room temperature. Slice peppers, onion, zucchini, and olives into 1-inch square chunks and toss together in a mixing bowl. Set aside.

Cut eggplant in half, scoop out flesh with a spoon and drain over a colander, pressing flesh down lightly with the spoon to remove excess water. Transfer eggplant to a food processor fitted with a standard blade.

Add remaining Baba Ghanoush ingredients to food processor, puree until smooth and transfer mixture to a separate small bowl. Set aside at room temperature until ready to use.

Divide dough ball in half. Roll out each dough half to a 6-to 8-inch diameter. Spray 1 side of each evenly with cooking spray. Carefully place piece of dough onto grill, sprayed-side-down. Grill for 1 to 3 minutes or until bottom of dough is lightly charred. Using a pizza pan and a grill spatula, carefully slide crust from grill onto pan and transport crust to your counter. Spray un-grilled side crust with cooking spray and flip dough over on pan, now grilled-side-up. Repeat with second piece of dough, placing both pizzas onto pan grilled-side-up.

Spread 1/3 cup Baba Ghanoush evenly onto each pizza crust, almost to the edge. Drain liquid from grilled vegetables and distribute veggies onto both pizzas, diving evenly. Leaving pizzas on pan, place pan onto grill, close lid and grill for about 2 to 3 minutes, until bottom of pizzas are crisp and lightly charred.

Remove from grill, carefully slice each pizza into 4 wedges and serve immediately with a dollop of remaining Baba Ghanoush on each slice (about ½ tsp. per slice).

SERVES

8 SLICES, 2 PIZZAS

BBQ-Chicken Pizza

INGREDIENTS

1 large whole wheat tortilla

2 ½ Tbsp. barbecue sauce

½ cup fat-free cheddar cheese

2/3 cup grilled chicken breast, chopped

¼ cup red onion

2 tsp. fresh cilantro leaves, chopped

Preheat the oven to 400 degrees

Place the tortilla on a small nonstick baking sheet. Bake for 4-5 minutes per side, or until crisp. If air bubbles form, poke them with a fork, then press out the air with a spatula or oven mitt. Remove the sheet from the oven. Top the tortilla evenly in layers with the sauce, cheese, chicken, onion, and cilantro. Bake for 2-4 minutes, or until the cheese is completely melted. Slice into 8 wedges. Serve immediately.

Chicken Alfredo Pizza

INGREDIENTS

1 package Simply Organic (brand) alfredo mix (use almond or rice milk and low-fat parmesan cheese for mix)

100% Whole Wheat prepared pizza crust Boboli (brand)

2 Tbsp. extra-virgin olive oil

2 cups fat-free mozzarella cheese

2-3 boneless, skinless chicken breasts, grilled and diced

Low fat parmesan cheese

Red onion

Tomatoes, diced

Peppers, color of your choice

Mushrooms

Preheat the oven to temperature indicated on the pizza crust package.

Cook alfredo mix as directed on package; allow to cool and slightly thicken.

Spread olive oil on crust. Spread alfredo mix on crust. Add diced grilled chicken pieces and toppings as desired. Sprinkle mozzarella cheese evenly over pizza.

Bake as directed on pizza crust package.

Sausage Pizza

INGREDIENTS

Olive oil spray

1 cup sweet onion strips

1 cup sliced button mushrooms

¾ cup green bell pepper, strips

4 oz. 96% lean ground beef or ground turkey

2 ½ oz. fresh turkey or chicken Italian sausage, sliced

16 oz. fresh or frozen whole wheat pizza dough, defrosted, if necessary or 100% whole wheat prepared pizza crust Boboli (brand)

¾ cup low-fat, low sodium pizza sauce from a jar

1 ½ cups shredded fat-free mozzarella cheese

8 slices turkey pepperoni

2 Tbsp. kalamata olives, pitted and sliced

1 tsp. oregano

1 ½ Tbsp. crushed red pepper flakes

Preheat oven to 450 degrees.

Heat a medium nonstick frying pan over medium heat and lightly mist with spray. Add onions, mushrooms, and peppers. Cook about 6-8 minutes, until vegetables are tender and just barely starting to brown. Remove pan contents into another dish.

Turn heat to medium-high and return pan to heat. When hot, add ground beef and sausage. Cook, stirring occasionally, breaking beef into hearty chunks until just barely pink, about 1-2 minutes.

Remove and turn off heat.

In a 12- or 14-inch nonstick pizza pan, using a rolling pin and flour, gently press dough to 12-inch diameter, being careful not to create any holes (crust will be crispier if pan is dark gray or black). If dough tears, patch it. Then, using a fork, poke dough about 20 times, evenly spreading out the holes. Bake for 4 minutes.

Spoon sauce in center of dough, then spread evenly to cover all but the outer inch. Sprinkle cheese evenly over sauce. Then top evenly with pepperoni, sausage mixture, vegetable mixture, then olives.

Sprinkle with oregano and red pepper flakes. Bake an additional 12-15 minutes or until crust is lightly browned (but before the cheese browns). Remove. Let stand for 5 minutes. Then transfer to cutting board and slice into 8 slices.

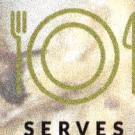

SERVES
4

Eggplant Pizza

INGREDIENTS

100% Whole Wheat prepared pizza crust Boboli (brand)

¾ cup low-fat, low-sodium marinara sauce

¾ cup fat-free mozzarella cheese

½ cup fat-free or reduced-fat ricotta cheese

3 plum tomatoes

¾ lb. eggplant

1 ½ Tbsp. reduced-fat parmesan cheese

2 Tbsp. basil leaves

Ground pepper, to taste

Preheat oven at 450 degrees.

Spread marinara sauce on pizza crust, and then sprinkle with mozzarella cheese.

Dollop ricotta cheese over pizza, and top with sliced fresh plum tomatoes and broiled sliced eggplant

Sprinkle finely grated parmesan cheese, and bake for 10-12 minutes or until golden brown. Sprinkle with fresh basil leaves, cut into 5 slices, and serve.

SERVES 5

Potato & Bacon Pizza

INGREDIENTS

100% Whole Wheat prepared pizza crust Boboli (brand)

¾ cup fontina cheese, coarsely shredded

2 tsp. rosemary, finely chopped

½ lb. new potatoes, thinly sliced

4 slices turkey bacon, cooked and crumbled

2 Tbsp. reduced-fat parmesan cheese, finely grated

Preheat oven at 450 degrees.

Sprinkle ¾ cup coarsely shredded fontina cheese and finely chopped rosemary on pizza crust. Then top with thinly sliced new potatoes; chopped rosemary; 4 slices turkey bacon, cooked and crumbled; and finely grated parmesan cheese.

Bake for 12 minutes or until golden brown. Cut into 5 slices, and serve.

SERVES 5

Alaskan Salmon Pizza

INGREDIENTS

100% Whole Wheat prepared pizza crust Boboli (brand)

¾ cup fat-free cream cheese

2 Tbsp. fresh dill, chopped

1 ½ Tbsp. lemon juice

3 oz. smoked salmon, sliced

1 Tbsp. capers

¼ cup red onion, sliced

Ground pepper, to taste

Preheat oven at 450 degrees.

Combine ¾ cup cream cheese with fresh dill and lemon juice. Spread mixture on crust. Top with sliced smoked salmon, capers, and red onion.

Bake for 10-12 minutes or until crust is crisp.

Garnish with fresh dill. Cut into 5 slices; serve.

SERVES

5

Italian Pizza

INGREDIENTS

100% Whole Wheat prepared pizza crust Boboli (brand)

¾ cup fat-free mozzarella cheese

½ cup reduced-fat ricotta cheese

1/3 cup reduced-fat goat cheese, crumbled

2 Tbsp. reduced-fat parmesan cheese, grated

2 ½ Tbsp. fresh thyme

½ cup fresh Roma tomatoes

Preheat oven at 450 degrees.

Sprinkle mozzarella cheese, dollop ricotta cheese, and crumbled goat cheese on pizza crust.

Top with grated Parmesan cheese and fresh thyme.

Then bake for 12-15 minutes or until golden brown. Cut into 5 slices; serve.

SERVES

5

Mushroom Thin-Crust Pizza

INGREDIENTS

Olive oil cooking spray

2 Tbsp. garlic, minced

2 ¼ cups cremini mushrooms, thinly sliced

3 tsp. rosemary sprigs, finely chopped, divided

1 lb. package store-bought whole wheat pizza dough

1 tsp. + 1 Tbsp. extra-virgin olive oil, divided

2 medium plum tomatoes, diced

2 oz. reduced-fat goat cheese, crumbled

3 Tbsp. white balsamic vinegar

¼ medium radicchio, thinly sliced and soaked in cold water for 30 minutes

2 cups baby arugula

Preheat oven to 475 degrees.

Coat a large sauté pan with cooking spray and set over medium-high heat. Add garlic and mushrooms and sauté for 4 to 6 minutes or until tender, light golden brown in color and no liquid remains in pan.

Transfer garlic-mushroom mixture to a bowl, season with 1 tsp. rosemary and mix well. Set aside at room temperature.

Line a large baking sheet with parchment paper and sprinkle with cornmeal.

Roll out pizza dough into a rectangular shape, as thin as possible, about 12 inches x 16 inches in size.

Transfer dough onto baking sheet and brush with 1 tsp. oil. Top pizza with remaining rosemary, tomatoes, and cheese and season with salt and pepper. Place pan into oven and bake for 8 to 10 minutes, until crust is golden brown and crisp. Remove from oven and slice crust in half lengthwise, then cut each half into 6 pieces.

While pizza is baking, prepare dressing: In a small bowl, whisk remaining 1 Tbsp.. oil into vinegar.

Drain radicchio well and place into a large bowl. Add arugula and dressing to radicchio and toss well, seasoning with salt and pepper.

Top each pizza slice with radicchio salad and garlic-mushroom mixture, dividing evenly. Serve immediately.

SERVES

6

Margherita Pizza

INGREDIENTS

100% Whole Wheat prepared pizza crust Boboli (brand)

¾ cup marinara sauce (add some red pepper flakes for a little kick) or arrabiata sauce

½ cup fat-free smoked mozzarella cheese, shredded

¼ cup fat-free mozzarella cheese, shredded

2 ½ Tbsp. fresh basil, chopped

1 tsp. red pepper flakes

Preheat oven at 450 degrees.

Spread ¾ cup marinara or arrabiata sauce on pizza crust, then sprinkle both cheeses and red pepper flakes.

Bake for 12 minutes or until golden brown. Top with chopped fresh basil. Cut into 5 slices; serve.

SERVES

5

Spicy Mexican Rancheros

INGREDIENTS

Ranchero Sauce Ingredients:

1 ½ tsp. extra-virgin olive oil

1 small yellow onion, chopped

1 ½ Tbsp. garlic, chopped

1-14oz. can diced fire roasted tomatoes, no salt added

1 Tbsp. Frank Hot Sauce

1 tsp. ground cumin

½ tsp. dried oregano

Ground pepper, to taste

½ tsp. dried chipotle powder

½ tsp. red pepper flakes

¼ cup fresh cilantro, chopped

For each serving of Rancheros:

1 corn tortilla or whole wheat tortilla

2 Tbsp. fat-free refried beans

2 egg whites

Garnish:

1 ½ Tbsp. shredded fat-free cheddar cheese

cilantro

Instructions for Sauce:

Heat the oil in a nonstick skillet. Add the onion and cook for about 5 minutes, or until softened. Add the garlic and cook for about 1 minute longer, but don't allow the garlic to brown.

Add the tomatoes, cumin, oregano, pepper, and chipotle powder, and cook for a few minutes longer.

Carefully transfer the sauce to the jar of a blender or the bowl of a food processor and blend or process briefly. The finished sauce should be a bit chunky. Stir in the cilantro.

To make on serving of Huevos Rancheros:

Warm the tortilla and refried beans and set aside.

Coat a small nonstick skillet with cooking spray. Add the egg whites and cook until nearly set or about 2 minutes. Turn the eggs with a silicone spatula and cook for about 1 minute longer.

Place the tortilla on a plate and top it with the refried beans. Place the cooked egg whites on the beans.

Top with ½ cup hot Ranchero Sauce and garnish with cheese and cilantro.

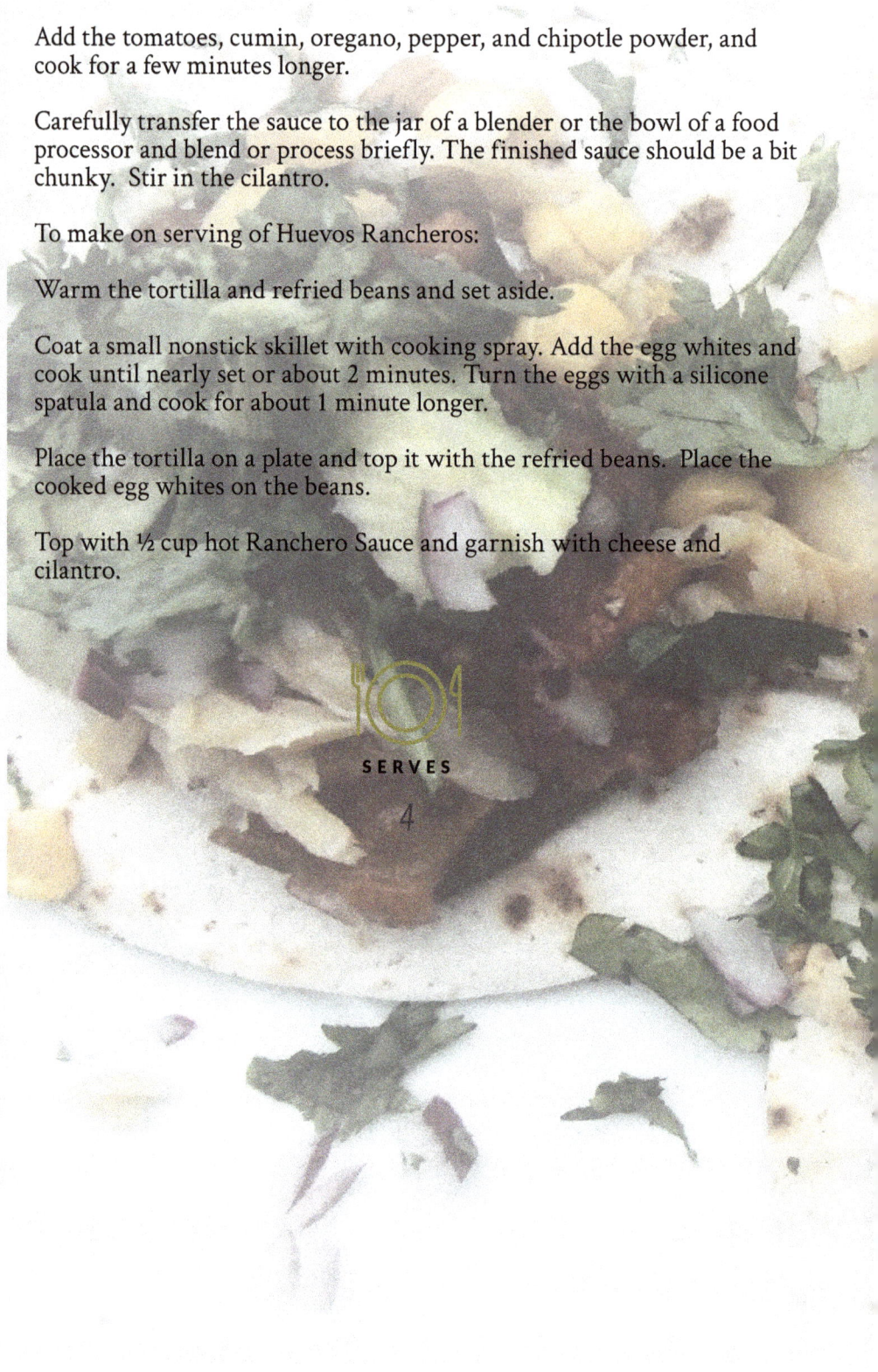

SERVES

4

Black Bean Tostadas

INGREDIENTS

1 cup cooked black beans

1 tsp. chipotle pepper, minced

1 tsp. cumin

½ tsp. chili powder

½ tsp. red pepper flakes

2 tsp. fresh lime juice, divided

½ cup frozen corn kernels, thawed

1 tostada shell

1 oz. fat-free cheddar cheese

1 cup frisee, washed, dried, and torn

1 cup cherry tomatoes, halved

In a food processor or medium bowl, puree or mash beans. Add chipotle, cumin, chili powder, red pepper flakes, and 1 tsp. lime juice, and mix well. Add bean mixture to a small pan and warm gently, stirring, over medium-low heat.

Warm corn in another small pan over medium-low heat.

Divide bean mixture between 2 halves of sandwich thin, spreading evenly. Place halves, bean-side up, on a plate. Top with cheese and corn, dividing evenly. Sprinkle remaining 1 tsp. lime juice over frisee, then scatter evenly over halves. Garnish with tomatoes and serve immediately.

Healthy Tostadas

INGREDIENTS

8 tostada shells

1 bag prewashed romaine lettuce, shredded

2 medium Roma tomatoes, diced

1-15.5oz can reduced-sodium or unsalted black beans, drained and rinsed

¾ cup shredded fat-free or reduced-fat Monterey Jack cheese

4 green onions, thinly sliced

½ cup salsa

½ cup corn

Yogurt-Onion Sauce Ingredients:

1 small red onion, finely diced

1 Tbsp. lime juice

1 cup plain fat-free yogurt

2 Tbsp. minced garlic

1 Tbsp. Tabasco

Make the Yogurt-Onion Sauce first: Place red onion in a bowl and sprinkle with a bit of salt; mix well with fingers and let rest for 5 minutes. In a small bowl, stir remaining sauce ingredients together. When the onion is translucent and watery, rinse well in a colander and add to the yogurt mixture. Stir well and set aside.

Place 2 tostada shells on each plate; alternatively, arrange shells around the perimeter of a large serving platter. Place shredded lettuce in center of shells.

Top greens with diced tomatoes, black beans, and corn, dividing them evenly. Sprinkle cheese on beans and top with green onions. Top each with a dollop of salsa and Yogurt-Onion Sauce.

SERVES

4

Portobello & Cheese Quesadillas

INGREDIENTS

4 large Portobello mushroom caps

¼ cup fat free parmesan cheese

1 tsp. extra-virgin olive oil

4 whole wheat tortillas

½ cup fat-free mozzarella cheese, thinly sliced

8 fresh basil leaves, torn by hand

3 roasted red bell peppers, thinly sliced

Ground pepper, to taste

Build a fire in a charcoal grill, letting the coals burn down until covered with white ash or preheat a gas grill to medium. If using a grill pan, preheat the pan briefly over medium-high heat.

Brush each mushroom cap with olive oil, season them with a pinch of salt, and grill until grill marks form and the mushrooms are tender, 4 to 5 minutes per side. Transfer the mushrooms to a plate and let cool. Leave the heat going. When cool enough to handle, thinly slice the mushrooms.

Arrange the mushroom slices over the bottom half of each wrap. Top with the mozzarella, basil, pepper, and roasted pepper slices. Fold the top of the wraps over the filling.

Grill the wraps just long enough to warm the filling through and melt the cheese so it holds the wraps together, about 1 minute per side.

Put 1 quesadilla on each of 4 plates and serve.

SERVES

4

Must Have Healthy Enchiladas

INGREDIENTS

2 boneless, skinless chicken breasts, cooked and shredded

1 cup cooked brown rice

1 can chili, black or fat free refried beans

½ cup salsa

6-100% whole wheat tortillas

1 cup fat-free cottage cheese

1 can enchilada sauce

½ pepper, any color of your choice

1 large jalapeno, sliced with seeds

½ red onion

Preheat oven to 350 degrees.

In a large bowl mix chicken, rice, beans, salsa, cottage cheese, peppers, jalapeno, and red onions.

Divide equally between 6 tortillas and place in sprayed baking dish.

Top with enchilada sauce, cover with foil. Place in oven for 30 minutes, uncover to 15 additional minutes. Serve with lettuce, tomato, avocado, and salsa.

SERVES

6

Sweet Fire Shrimp Tacos

INGREDIENTS

1 cup fresh or frozen pitted red cherries

2 jalapeno peppers, cut in half

2 tsp. ginger, minced

4 tsp. organic honey or Stevia

24 large raw shrimp, remove tails and shell

1 Tbsp. extra-virgin olive oil

8-100% whole wheat corn soft taco shells

1 small head radicchio, thinly sliced

4 large carrots, peeled and grated

4 Tbsp. cilantro leaves

Place cherries, jalapeno, ginger, and honey/Stevia in a mini chopper or blender along with ¼ cup water. Blend until smooth (there may be very small bits of cherry).

Heat a large skillet over high heat. Add oil and shrimp and cook for 2 to 3 minutes, turning occasionally, until shrimp are pink on the outside but not cooked through. Reduce heat to medium and carefully add cherry mixture. Simmer for about 2 minutes, until sauce reduces slightly and shrimp are cooked through.

-Preheat an oven or toaster oven to 400 degrees and warm taco shells for 2 minutes. Spoon 3 shrimp and 1 Tbsp. cherry sauce into each taco and top with 2 Tbsp. each radicchio and carrots. Garnish with cilantro, if desired. Serve immediately.

It's **common** to mistake thirst for hunger, so staying well hydrated will also help you make healthier food choices.

Chili Chicken Tacos

INGREDIENTS

12 oz chicken breast (organic), cut in strips

1 Tbsp. chili powder

4 whole wheat tortillas

3 cups shredded romaine lettuce

2 Roma tomatoes, diced

½ red onion, sliced

1 lime

1 avocado, pitted and peeled

¼ cup cottage cheese

2 Tbsp. chopped cilantro leaves

In a skillet, cook chicken on medium-high heat. Season chicken with chili powder. Cook until chicken is no longer pink in the middle. Then remove from heat.

In a blender, blend avocado, cottage cheese and cilantro until smooth.

Warm tortillas in microwave or on skillet (read directions on package). Add lettuce, tomatoes, onion, chicken, and avocado cream. Squeeze a fresh lime over the top before serving for added flavor.

The Healthier Banana Bread

INGREDIENTS

3 egg whites

3 ripe bananas, mashed

½ cup unsweetened applesauce

¾ cup Stevia

2 cups 100% whole wheat flour

1 tsp. baking powder

2 Tbsp. cinnamon

½ cup almonds, chopped or slivered (optional)

Preheat oven to 325 degrees.

In a medium bowl, beat the egg whites, and add the remaining wet ingredients; mix thoroughly.

In another bowl, mix the dry ingredients. Then lightly blend all of the ingredients together, and pour the mixture into a loaf pan.

Bake for 50 minutes or until a toothpick comes out dry. Let the loaf stand in the pan for 10 minutes, then slice and serve.

Tasty Apple Zucchini Bread

INGREDIENTS

Olive oil cooking spray

1 ¼ cups 100% whole wheat flour

¼ cup spelt flour

2 tsp. baking powder

½ tsp. baking soda

1 Tbsp. cinnamon

1 Gala apple, grated

1 zucchini, grated

1 egg

½ cup fat-free plain Greek yogurt

¼ cup raw honey, Stevia, or agave nectar

Preheat oven to 350 degrees. Mist an 8 x 4-inch or 9 x 5-inch loaf pan with cooking spray.

In a large bowl, whisk together flours, baking powder, baking soda, and cinnamon; set aside.

In a separate bowl, whisk together apple, zucchini, egg, yogurt, and honey, Stevia, or agave nectar.

Add wet ingredients to dry ingredients and fold until just combined. Spread batter into prepared pan and bake until golden brown, 40 to 45 minutes.

SERVES

10

Carrot Cake Bread

INGREDIENTS

1 lb. sweet carrots, peeled and grated

1 ¼ cups 100% whole wheat flour

1 ¼ cups cornmeal

¼ cup flax meal

1 ½ tsp. baking powder

2 tsp. cinnamon

3 egg whites

1 egg yolk

2 Tbsp. extra-virgin olive oil

½ cup organic honey, Stevia, or agave nectar

¾ cup almond or rice milk

¼ cup raisins and ¼ unsweetened cranberries

Olive oil cooking spray

Preheat oven to 375 degrees.

In a small saucepan place carrots and enough water to just cover them. Bring to a boil and cook for 5 minutes. Remove from heat, drain, and let cool.

In a medium mixing bowl place dry ingredients: flour, cornmeal, salt, flax meal, baking powder, and cinnamon.

In another bowl, whip egg whites until stiff.

In small bowl put egg yolk, oil, honey, and milk. Mix well. Add to dry ingredients and mix until just combined. Add whipped egg whites and fold until just combined. Add dried fruits and cooked carrots and mix until just combined. Do not over-mix or loaf will get hard.

Prepare a 5" x 9" loaf pan with cooking spray. Pour batter into loaf pan and bake for 60 minutes or until cake tester comes out clean. Makes 10 servings, more or less, depending how thick you slice the bread.

SERVES

10

Moms Healthy Granola

INGREDIENTS

1 cup organic rye flakes

1 cup organic oat flakes

1 cup organic wheat flakes

1 cup raw, sliced, unsalted almonds

½ cup unsalted sunflower seeds

¼ cup sesame seeds & ¼ Chia seeds

any other unsalted nuts of choice

½ cup no sugar added dried fruit

Coating Mixture Ingredients:

½ tsp. cinnamon

¼ cup extra-virgin olive oil

1 tsp. vanilla extract

¼ cup organic honey or Stevia

Preheat oven to 300 degrees. In a large bowl mix all dry ingredients until evenly distributed. Set aside.

Meanwhile, in a small saucepan, place all coating mixture ingredients. Gently warm contents and stir until honey is dissolved.

Pour liquid coating mixture over dry ingredients in mixing bowl. Using a large wooden spoon or clean bare hands, mix well until all ingredients are coated.

Spread granola onto a large cookie sheet lined with parchment paper.

Baking time is 40 minutes, but you can't walk away from the oven. You need to stir the granola every so often with a wooden spoon so everything gets nicely toasted.

Transfer baked granola to a cooking rack and sprinkle with raisins and cranberries (or other no sugar added dried fruit). Let cool completely. When cool, transfer to an airtight container. Keeps in your cereal cupboard for one week. You can freeze it too.

Healthy Tortilla Chips

INGREDIENTS

6-inch unsalted corn tortillas or 100% whole wheat tortillas

Olive oil cooking spray

Cayenne pepper or mild chili powder, to taste

Chile powder, to taste

Ground black pepper, to taste

Preheat oven to 400 degrees. Cut tortillas into quarters, lightly mist both sides with cooking spray and arrange in a single layer on 2 baking sheets. Dust tops with cayenne pepper and chili powder.

Amount will depend how much spice you can handle. Bake in oven for 5 to 6 minutes per side or until crisp and lightly browned. Chips will continue to crisp slightly as they cool. Serve immediately or cool completely and store in an airtight container for up to 8 hours.

Healthy Wild Rice

INGREDIENTS

1 ¼ cups water

3 cups certified organic, low-sodium chicken broth

1 ½ cups uncooked wild rice

1 Tbsp. extra-virgin olive oil

3 cups sliced mushrooms

1 cup chopped green onions

½ cup chopped fresh parsley

1/3 cup chopped pecans, toasted (optional)

¾ tsp. poultry seasoning

1 tsp. freshly ground pepper

Olive oil cooking spray

Bring water and broth to a boil in a medium saucepan.

Add wild rice; cover, reduce heat, and simmer 1 hour or until tender. Drain any excess liquid.

Preheat oven to 325 degrees

Put olive oil in a large, nonstick skillet over medium-high heat, then add mushrooms and onions; sauté until tender

Remove from heat; stir in parsley and next 4 ingredients.

Combine rice and mushroom mixture in a 2-quart casserole, coated with nonfat cooking spray.

Cover and bake at 325 degrees for 25 minutes.

SERVES

8

Louisiana Dirty Rice & Red Beans

INGREDIENTS

1 cup brown rice

7 oz. deli-fresh smoked lean turkey sausage

Olive oil cooking spray

1 medium yellow onion, diced

1 green bell pepper, cored, seeded, and diced

2 Tbsp. garlic, minced

8 oz. dried red beans, soaked overnight in water in a covered pot

1 bay leaf

2 Roma tomatoes, finely chopped

1 ½ tsp. Cajun seasoning

4 Tbsp. fresh cilantro

1 tsp. Tabasco sauce

Cook brown rice according to package directions. Remove from heat and set aside.

In a medium-size port, cover sausage with about 3 inches of water. Bring to a boil, then allow to boil for 10 minutes. Remove from heat, drain and let cool for 5 minutes before slicing sausage.

Heat a large pot over medium-high heat. Mist with cooking spray and add onion, green pepper, garlic, and Tabasco sauce. Sauté for about 5 minutes or until vegetables are cooked through. Drain soaked beans and rinse with cold water. Add beans, bay leaf, and 3 cups water to pot with vegetables. Bring to a boil, then let boil for 20 minutes before reducing heat to medium-low. Cook until beans are soft, stirring occasionally and adding more water as it evaporates, about 2 hours. When beans are cooked through and water has reduced to less than 1 cup, add tomatoes and cook for at least 15 more minutes.

Remove bay leaf. Stir in Cajun seasoning, cooked rice, and sausage and cook for about 10 minutes.

Garnish with cilantro before serving.

***If opting to use canned beans verses dried beans, you will only need to warm them up for about 5 to 10 minutes instead of cooking them for 2 hours. And, you can reduce the water for 3 cups to ½ cup.

SERVES

6

Roasted Tomato & Shrimp Orzo

INGREDIENTS

1 pt. grape tomatoes or sun-dried tomatoes

3 tsp. extra-virgin olive oil

8 oz. or 1 ¼ cup whole-wheat orzo

1 can (15 to 19 oz.) white kidney beans/cannellini, rinsed and drained

12 oz. medium peeled and deveined shrimp

1-6 oz. bag baby spinach

2 oz. fat-free feta cheese

¼ tsp. ground black pepper

1 tsp. basil leaves

¼ cup packed fresh dill, chopped, plus additional springs for garnish, or to taste

Preheat oven to 450 degrees. Line 15 ½" by 10 1/2 "jelly-roll pan with foil. In prepared pan, combine tomatoes, 2 Tbsp. oil, and ¼ tsp. freshly ground black pepper. Roast 15 minutes or until tomatoes begin to collapse.

Meanwhile, heat covered 4-quart saucepan of water to boiling on high. Cook orzo as label directs; drain and return to pot.

In medium bowl, toss beans, shrimp, ¼ tsp. freshly ground black pepper, and remaining 1 tsp. olive oil. Add to tomato mixture; stir to combine. Spread in single layer and roast 5 minutes longer or until shrimp are opaque throughout.

Add spinach to orzo in pot; toss to wilt. Stir in shrimp mixture, feta, basil leave, and dill. Transfer to shallow bowls, garnish with dill springs.

SERVES

4

Quinoa Greek Chicken Feta Salad

INGREDIENTS

1 cup quinoa

2 tsp. extra-virgin olive oil

3 Tbsp. cloves garlic, minced

2 cups fresh spinach

2 oz. fat-free feta cheese

2 cups certified organic, low-sodium chicken broth

2 boneless, skinless chicken breasts

Rinse quinoa, add broth, and boil.

Reduce heat, cover to simmer 10-15 minutes until water is absorbed.

Cook garlic in olive oil. Then add quinoa when done.

Add spinach and once it starts to wilt add the rest of the ingredients.

Chicken Wild Rice Casserole

INGREDIENTS

4- 6oz. package wild long-grain rice with seasonings

14 oz. can low-sodium, low-fat chicken broth

1 can low-fat, low-sodium cream of chicken soup

1 cup almond or rice milk

1 lb. chicken breasts, sliced

1 can sliced water chestnuts, drained

2/3 cup plain protein powder

Paprika

½ tsp. cumin

Pour rice into a Crock-Pot. In a medium bowl, whisk chicken broth, soup, and milk together. Pour half of the mixture over rice and stir.

Add chicken breasts and water chestnuts to Crock-Pot, then remaining soup mixture.

Cover and cook on low for 4-6 hours or until chicken is cooked through and rice is tender.

Just before serving, whisk protein powder into chicken and rice mixture, which will thicken the sauce.

Sprinkle with paprika and cumin, and serve.

SERVES

4

Left-Over Turkey Casserole

INGREDIENTS

2 cups cubed, cooked skinless turkey breasts

1 package (10 oz.) frozen peas

1 cup celery, chopped

3 Tbsp. green pepper, chopped

2 Tbsp. onion, chopped

1 can reduced-fat, reduced-sodium, condensed cream of chicken soup

1 cup shredded fat-free cheddar cheese

¼ cup almond or rice milk

2 Tbsp. low-sodium chicken broth

2 Tbsp. lemon juice

2 slices whole wheat bread, cubed

Preheat oven to 375 degrees. In a large bowl, combine the first six ingredients.

In a small saucepan, combine the soup, milk, ½ cup of cheese, broth, and lemon juice. Cook and stir over low heat until smooth and heated through. Pour over turkey mixture and toss to coat. Transfer mixture to a baking dish coated with nonstick spray and top with bread cubes.

Bake uncovered for 25 minutes. Sprinkle remaining ½ cup cheese on top and bake another 5 minutes or until cheese is melted.

SERVES

6

Cook's Green Bean Casserole

INGREDIENTS

3 Tbsp. extra-virgin olive oil, divided

1lb 99% lean ground turkey

1 sweet onion, divided

8 oz. mushrooms, chopped

1 Tbsp. onion powder

1 tsp. dried thyme

½ tsp. freshly ground pepper

2/3 cup whole wheat flour, divided

1 cup almond or rice milk

3 Tbsp. dry sherry

4 cups French-cut green beans

1/3 cup fat-free plain Greek yogurt

3 Tbsp. buttermilk powder

2 tsp. paprika

1 tsp. garlic powder

Preheat oven to 400 degrees. Coat a 2 ½-quart baking dish with cooking spray.

Cook lean turkey set aside.

Heat 1 Tbsp. oil in a large saucepan over medium heat. Add diced onion and cook, stirring often, until softened and slightly translucent, about 4 minutes. Stir in mushrooms, onion powder, thyme, and pepper. Cook, stirring often, until the mushroom juices are almost evaporated, 3 to 5 minutes. Sprinkle 1/3 cup flour over the vegetables, stir to coat. Add milk and sherry and bring to a simmer, stirring often. Stir in green beans and return to a simmer. Cook, stirring, until heated through about 1 minute. Stir in Greek yogurt and buttermilk powder. Transfer to the prepared baking dish and add turkey.

Whisk the remaining 1/3 cup flour, paprika, and garlic powder in a shallow dish. Add sliced onion; toss to coat. Heat the remaining 2 Tbsp. oil in large nonstick skillet over medium-high heat. Add the onion along with any remaining flour mixture and cook, turning once or twice, until golden and crispy, 4 to 5 minutes. Spread the onion topping over the casserole.

Bake the casserole until bubbling, about 15 minutes. Let cool for 5 minutes before serving.

SERVES

6

Chicken Whole-Wheat Rotini with Asparagus and Snap Peas

INGREDIENTS

1 package (13 ¼ ounce) 100% whole-wheat rotini

1lb chicken

8 oz. asparagus, cut into pieces

8oz. stringless snap peas

1 Tbsp. extra-virgin olive oil

1 small onion, chopped

1 lemon

½ cup freshly grated reduced-fat Pecorino Romano cheese

½ cup packed fresh basil leaves, thinly sliced

2 Tbsp. chives

Heat large covered saucepan of salted water on high to boiling. Add pasta and cook as label directs, adding asparagus and snap peas when 3 minutes of cooking time remain.

Meanwhile, in 10-inch nonstick skillet, heat oil on medium until hot. Cook chicken white on both sides and then and add onion and cook 10 to 12 minutes or until tender and browned. From lemon, grate 1 tsp. peel and squeeze 2 Tbsp. juice.

Reserve ½ cup pasta cooking water; drain pasta and vegetables. In large serving bowl, toss pasta and vegetables with cooking water, onion, lemon peel and juice, Romano, basil, and chives.

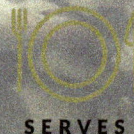

SERVES

4

Read food labels…… If you can't pronounce it, don't eat it!

Ginger Chicken Party Pasta

INGREDIENTS

8 oz. 100% whole-wheat angel hair pasta

2 tsp. peanut oil

1 tsp. garlic, minced

1 ½ Tbsp. fresh ginger, minced

1 lb. boneless, skinless chicken breasts, cut into long slices

¼ cup Braggs Amino Acid or tamari sauce

2 tsp. toasted sesame oil

3 Tbsp. fresh lime juice

¼ cup fresh cilantro, chopped

¼ cup scallions, chopped

Cook pasta according to package directions. Drain, reserving ¼ cup of cooking water.

Meanwhile, heat peanut oil in a large skillet over medium-high heat. Add garlic and ginger, and cook 1 minute. Add chicken and cook until golden brown on all sides, about 3 to 5 minutes. Add reserved cooking water, Braggs or tamari sauce, sesame oil, and lime juice. Bring to a simmer. Add pasta and cook 1 minute to heat through, stirring frequently.

Remove from heat and stir in cilantro and scallions.

SERVES

4

Sesame Pasta

INGREDIENTS

1 lb. 100% whole wheat spaghetti

½ cup Braggs Amino Acid or tamari sauce

2 Tbsp. sesame oil

2 Tbsp. extra-virgin olive oil

2 Tbsp. rice-wine vinegar

1 ½ Tbsp. lime juice

1 ½ tsp. red pepper flakes

½ cup scallions, sliced and divided

¼ cup fresh cilantro, chopped and divided

4 cups snow peas, sliced

1 red bell pepper, thinly sliced

½ cup toasted sesame seeds

Bring a large pot of water to a boil. Cook spaghetti until just tender, 9-11 minutes or according to package directions. Drain; rinse under cold water.

Meanwhile, Braggs or tamari sauce, sesame oil, olive oil, vinegar, lime juice, red pepper flakes, ¼ cup scallions, and 2 Tbsp. cilantro. Add noodles, snow peas, and bell pepper; toss to coat.

To serve, mix in sesame seeds and garnish with the remaining scallions and cilantro.

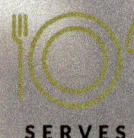

SERVES

8

Quinoa Pasta

INGREDIENTS

8 oz. Quinoa linguine

Olive oil cooking spray

6 large cloves garlic, finely chopped

1 large red heirloom tomato, diced into large chunks

2 cups packed fresh basil leaves

½ tsp. red pepper flakes

1 cup fat-free Greek yogurt or fat-free sour cream

1 oz. grated reduced-fat, low-sodium Parmigiano-Reggiano

2 Tbsp. toasted pine nuts, chopped

Bring large pot of water to boil. Cook pasta for about 7 minutes or follow package instructions.

Meanwhile, heat a medium sauté pan over medium-high heat. Spray pan with cooking spray and add half of the garlic. Sauté for 1 minute and add diced tomato. Sauté for about 3 minutes or until tomatoes are soft, but have not broken down too much.

Next, in the bowl of a food processor, combine: remaining 3 cloves chopped garlic with basil leaves, red pepper flakes, and fat-free Greek yogurt/sour cream. Puree until smooth.

When pasta is done cooking, drain and toss with creamy pesto sauce to coat; adjust seasonings, if necessary. Spoon tomato mixture on top of pasta and sprinkle with Parmigianino and pine nuts.

Serve.

SERVES

4

Vegetarian Spaghetti

INGREDIENTS

2 pints cherry tomatoes, halved

5 tsp. extra-virgin olive oil, divided

8 oz. 100% whole wheat spaghetti

1/3 cup fresh basil, chopped

½ cup ricotta cheese, crumbled

Preheat oven to 400 degrees.

Place tomatoes on a foil-lined baking sheet. Drizzle with 1 tsp. oil. Bake at 400 degrees for 20 minutes or until tomatoes collapse.

Cook pasta according to package directions. Drain pasta in a colander over a bowl, reserving 1/3 cup cooking liquid. Return pasta and served liquid to pan; stir in tomatoes, remaining 4 tsp. oil, basil, and cheese. Toss well. Serve immediately.

SERVES

4

Italian Chicken Pasta

INGREDIENTS

12 oz. cooked chicken breast

1 stalk celery, sliced

1 leek, white part with some green, rinsed and sliced

1 tsp. garlic, minced

1 cup low-sodium chicken or vegetable broth

1 Tbsp. no salt added tomato paste

½ cup sun-dried tomatoes, thinly sliced

1 tsp. rosemary

1 tsp. thyme

4 oz. dry whole wheat angel hair pasta

2 Tbsp. shredded Parmesan cheese

Olive oil cooking spray

Cut chicken into bite-size pieces and set aside; cover to keep warm. Boil water for pasta.

Coat a sauté pan with cooking spray and heat to medium-high. Add celery, leek, and garlic, and cook 4 to 5 minutes, until vegetables soften, adding a little broth to prevent burning, if necessary.

Add remaining broth and tomato paste; stir in sun-dried tomatoes and seasonings and bring to a simmer. Meanwhile, cook pasta according to package directions, drain and transfer to a serving bowl.

Stir chicken into vegetable mixture and heat through. Serve over pasta and top with Parmesan cheese.

Sweet & Sour Pasta

INGREDIENTS

1 lb. whole wheat linguine or spaghetti noodles

1 sweet onion, sliced

4 ½ cups broccoli florets

1 ½ lb. cleaned medium-size shrimp, peeled and deveined or chicken

1 bottle sweet and sour sauce (such as Kikkoman)

½ tsp. red pepper flakes

Bring a large pot of lightly salted water to a boil. Add linguine and cook as per package directions.

Drain.

Meanwhile, heat 2 Tbsp. oil in a 12-inch nonstick skillet over medium-high heat. Add onions and cook for 2 minutes. Add broccoli and continue to cook, stirring, and an additional 5 minutes. Add meat; season with ½ tsp. salt and ¼ tsp. black pepper. Cook and stir 3 to 5 minutes or until shrimp is no longer pink.

Stir in sweet and sour sauce, red pepper flakes, and linguine, tossing with tongs so that ingredients are well blended. Remove from heat; divide onto six plates. Serve immediately.

SERVES

6

Greek Pasta Salad

INGREDIENTS

1 lb. 100% whole wheat fusilli pasta noodles

7 oz. jar roasted pepper, drained and cut into bite-size

6 oz. jar marinated artichoke hearts, drained and cut into bite-size

½ cup crumbled herb fat-free feta cheese

¼ cup each sun-dried tomatoes, cut into strips,

¼ cup parsley, chopped

¼ cup olive oil

3 Tbsp. + 1 tsp. red wine vinegar

2 tsp. garlic, minced

Cook pasta in a large pot of water as package directs.

Meanwhile, put remaining ingredients in a large bowl; stir to combine.

Drain pasta. Rinse under cold water; drain well. Add to bowl; toss to mix and coat. Serve at room temperature.

SERVES

8

Thai Peanut Cold Noodle Salad

INGREDIENTS

½ lb. spaghetti or angel hair pasta

6 Tbsp. creamy peanut butter

3 Tbsp. rice vinegar

2 Tbsp. Braggs Amino Acid or tamari sauce

2 Tbsp. chili-garlic sauce or a dash of hot pepper sauce

½ almond or rice milk (almond milk may work a little better due to having a thicker consistency)

1 Tbsp. lime juice

1 Tbsp. grated fresh ginger

½ tsp. grated lime zest

1 Tbsp. extra-virgin olive oil

½ cup fresh cilantro, roughly chopped

¼ cup Vidalia onion, chopped

½ cup peapods, cut in half

1 ½ cup firmly packed broccoli florets

¼ cup salted peanuts, roughly chopped (optional)

Cook the pasta according to the package directions. Drain and rinse under cold running water.

Meanwhile combine the peanut butter, vinegar, Braggs or tamari sauce, chili-garlic sauce or hot pepper sauce, milk, lemon juice, ginger, and lime zest in a blender. With the motor running, slowly add the olive oil in a steady stream.

Return the pasta to the pot and toss with the dressing. Then add the onions, peapods, and broccoli and toss again. Garnish with the cilantro and peanuts (option). Serve immediately or cover and refrigerate for up to 3 hours.

If you're in the mood for salad rather than pasta, toss the Peanut Butter Dressing with shredded cabbage or lettuce, carrots, and cooked chicken.

SERVES

4

Vietnamese Pad Thai

INGREDIENTS

8 oz. rice noodles

2 Tbsp. no-salt-added tomato paste

1 Tbsp. tamarind paste

1 cup hot tap water

2 ½ Tbsp. agave nectar

3 Tbsp. Asian fish sauce

1 tsp. red chili flakes

1 Tbsp. refined safflower oil

2 tsp. garlic, minced

10 oz. extra-firm tofu, cubed

½ red onion, sliced

½ cup finely shredded red cabbage

4 green onions (green and white parts)

1 ½ cups bean sprouts

1 carrot, shredded

2 Roma tomatoes, diced

4 Tbsp. cilantro

2 Tbsp. roasted unsalted peanuts, chopped

4 to 8 lime wedges

Prepare noodles for stir-frying according to package directions. Drain and set aside.

In a medium bowl, whisk tomato paste and tamarind paste with 1 cup hot tap water. Stir in agave, fish sauce, and chili flakes. Set aside.

In a large wok or skillet over medium-high heat, combine oil and garlic and stir-fry just until garlic begins to brown, about 2 minutes. Add tofu and stir-fry for 1 minute. Add red onion and stir-fry for 30 seconds. Add cabbage and stir-fry for 30 seconds. Add noodles and sauce mixture and cook, stirring occasionally, until noodles are tender, about 3 minutes. Add green onions, bean sprouts, and carrot, and cook, stirring occasionally, until all ingredients are well combined and heated through.

Serve pad Thai topped with tomatoes, mint, cilantro, peanuts, and lime wedges.

SERVES

4

Protein Power Pad-Thai

INGREDIENTS

8 oz. rice noodles, flat (enough hot boiled water to cover noodles*)

1 Tbsp. extra-virgin olive oil

2 tsp. garlic

2 cups shredded Savoy cabbage

2 carrots, sliced thin

5 egg whites, lightly beaten

12 oz chicken or shrimp

3 cups bean sprouts

1 cup julienned green zucchini

1 cup green onions, chopped

1/3 cup fresh cilantro, chopped for garnish

* Reserve 2 Tbsp. noodle water

Sauce Ingredients:

3 Tbsp. rice wine vinegar or rice vinegar

¼ cup no salt added tomato paste

2 Tbsp. reserved noodle water

2 Tbsp. unsulfured molasses

2 Tbsp. Braggs Amino Acid or tamari sauce

Cover rice noodles with boiling water in a ceramic bowl. Cover and let stand for 20 minutes to soften noodles. Drain, reserving 2 Tbsp. noodle water.

In a small bowl, whisk together all sauce ingredients. Set aside.

Cook protein choice and set aside

In a large skillet, heat oil over medium heat. Stir in garlic, cabbage, and carrot. Stir-fry for 5 minutes.

Make a well in the middle of the pan and scramble the egg whites. Add noodles and sauce, and cook for 5 minutes. Add bean sprouts, zucchini, and green onions and cook a little longer to heat through.

Add protein back in and remove from heat and serve. Garnish each dish with chopped cilantro.

SERVES

8

Chicken Pasta

INGREDIENTS

1 Tbsp. garlic, minced

½ red onion, chopped

2 boneless, skinless chicken breasts, grilled and diced

1 yellow pepper

1 red pepper

1 broccoli floret, cut into small pieces

¼ cup parmesan cheese

1 box 100% whole wheat totini pasta

6 Tbsp. extra-virgin olive oil

Season with Mrs. Dash or 1 package Simply Organic (brand) alfredo mix (use almond or rice milk and reduced-fat parmesan cheese for mix)

Cook box of pasta separate.

Cook all other ingredients together and mix with pasta when done. Season with Mrs. Dash spices as desired or make alfredo sauce separately and combine.

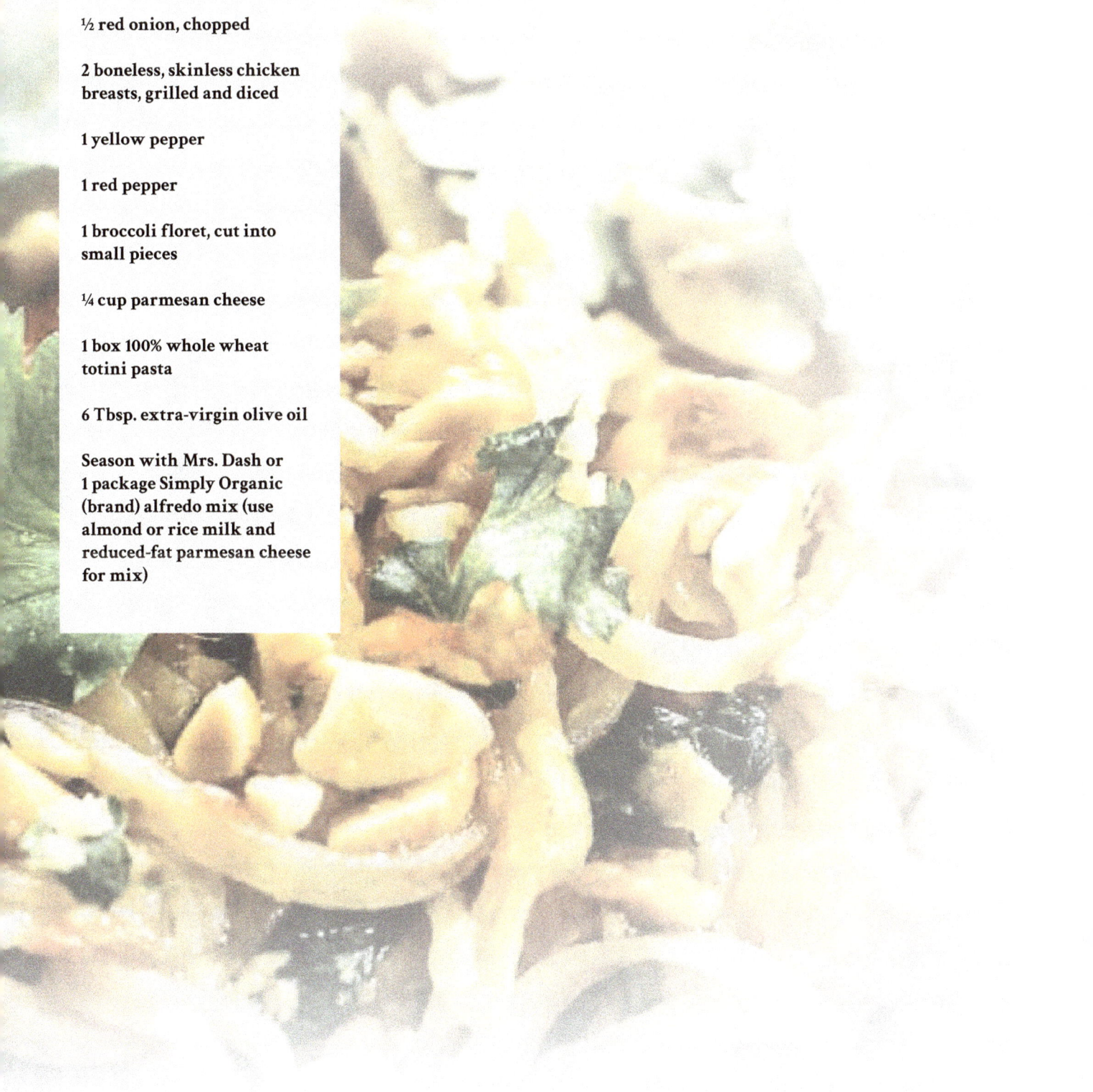

J R's Pestozini Penne

INGREDIENTS

1 package Pesto Chicken Sausages from Trader Joe's

1 box brown rice penne pasta

½ cup no salt added spaghetti sauce

1/3 yellow onion

1 Tbsp. red curry paste

½ Tbsp. Frank's hot sauce

¼ Tbsp. Frank's hot buffalo sauce

½ Tbsp. rice vinegar

4 Tbsp. extra-virgin olive oil

¼ jar roasted red pepper tapenade from Trader Joe's

¼ jar red pepper spread with eggplant and garlic from Trader Joe's

¼ cup sundried tomatoes

Cook pasta according to the direction on the package.

Cook all the other ingredients together (meat, vegetables, and sauces) for about 4-5 minutes on medium heat, then mix in with pasta.

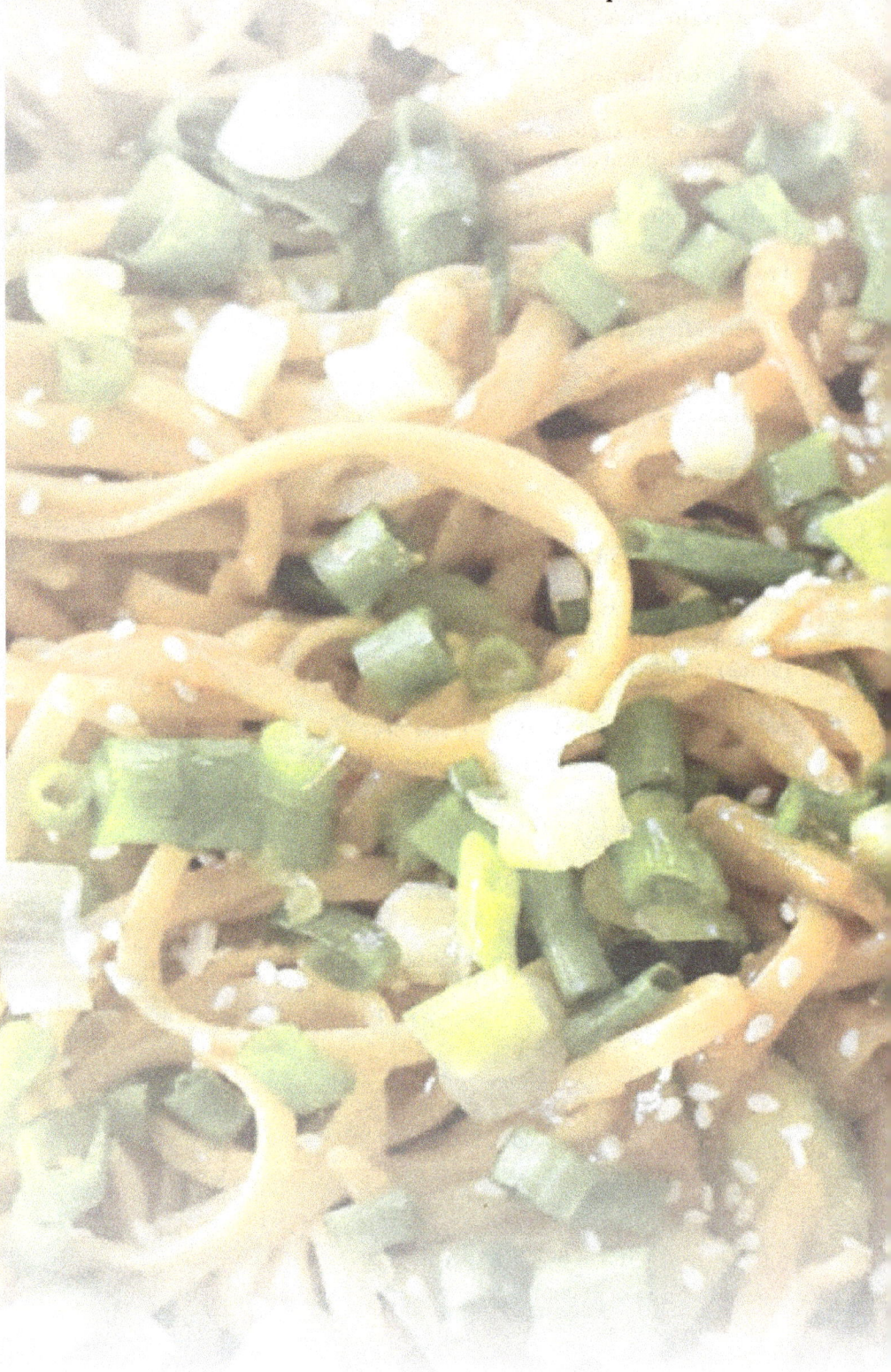

Spicy Noodles

INGREDIENTS

1 Tbsp. dark sesame oil, divided

1 Tbsp. grated peeled fresh ginger

1 Tbsp. garlic, minced

2 cups roasted skinless, boneless chicken breasts, chopped

½ cup green onions, chopped

¼ cup fresh cilantro, chopped

1 tsp. red pepper flakes

4 Tbsp. Braggs Amino Acid or tamari sauce

2 Tbsp. rice vinegar

2 Tbsp. hoisin sauce

2 Tbsp. ground fresh chili paste

1 package thin rice sticks

2 Tbsp. dry-roasted peanuts, chopped

Heat 2 tsp. oil in a small skillet over medium-high heat. Add ginger and garlic to pan; cook 45 seconds, stirring constantly. Place in a large bowl. Stir in remaining 1 tsp. oil, chicken, and next 7 ingredients (through chili paste).

Cook noodles according to package directions. Drain and rinse under cold water; drain. Cut noodles into smaller pieces. Add noodles to bowl; toss well to coat. Sprinkle with peanuts.

SERVES

4

Sun-Dried-Tomato and Pesto Risotto

INGREDIENTS

5 cups canned low-sodium chicken broth

1 cup water

3 Tbsp. extra-virgin olive oil

1 Vidalia onion, chopped

2 cups Arborio rice

½ cup dry white wine

¾ cup dry-packed sun-dried tomatoes, chopped

3 Tbsp. store-bought or homemade pesto

¼ cup grated reduced-fat Parmesan, more for serving

Pine nuts, for garnish

In a medium saucepan, bring the broth and water to a simmer. In a large pot, heat the oil over moderately low heat. Add the onion and cook, stirring occasionally, until translucent, about 5 minutes.

Add the rice to the pot and stir until it begins to turn opaque, about 2 minutes. Add the wine and cook, stirring frequently, until all the wine has been absorbed.

Add the sun-dried tomatoes and about ½ cup of the simmering broth to the rice and cook, stirring frequently, until the broth has been completely absorbed. The rice and broth should bubble gently; adjust the heat as needed. Continue cooking the rice, adding broth ½ cup at a time and allowing the rice to absorb the broth before adding the net ½ cup. Cook the rice in this way until tender, 25-30 minutes in all. The broth that hasn't been absorbed should be thickened by the starch from the rice. You may not need to use all the liquid, or you may need more broth or some water.

Stir in the pesto, and Parmesan. Serve the risotto with additional Parmesan and pine nuts, if desired.

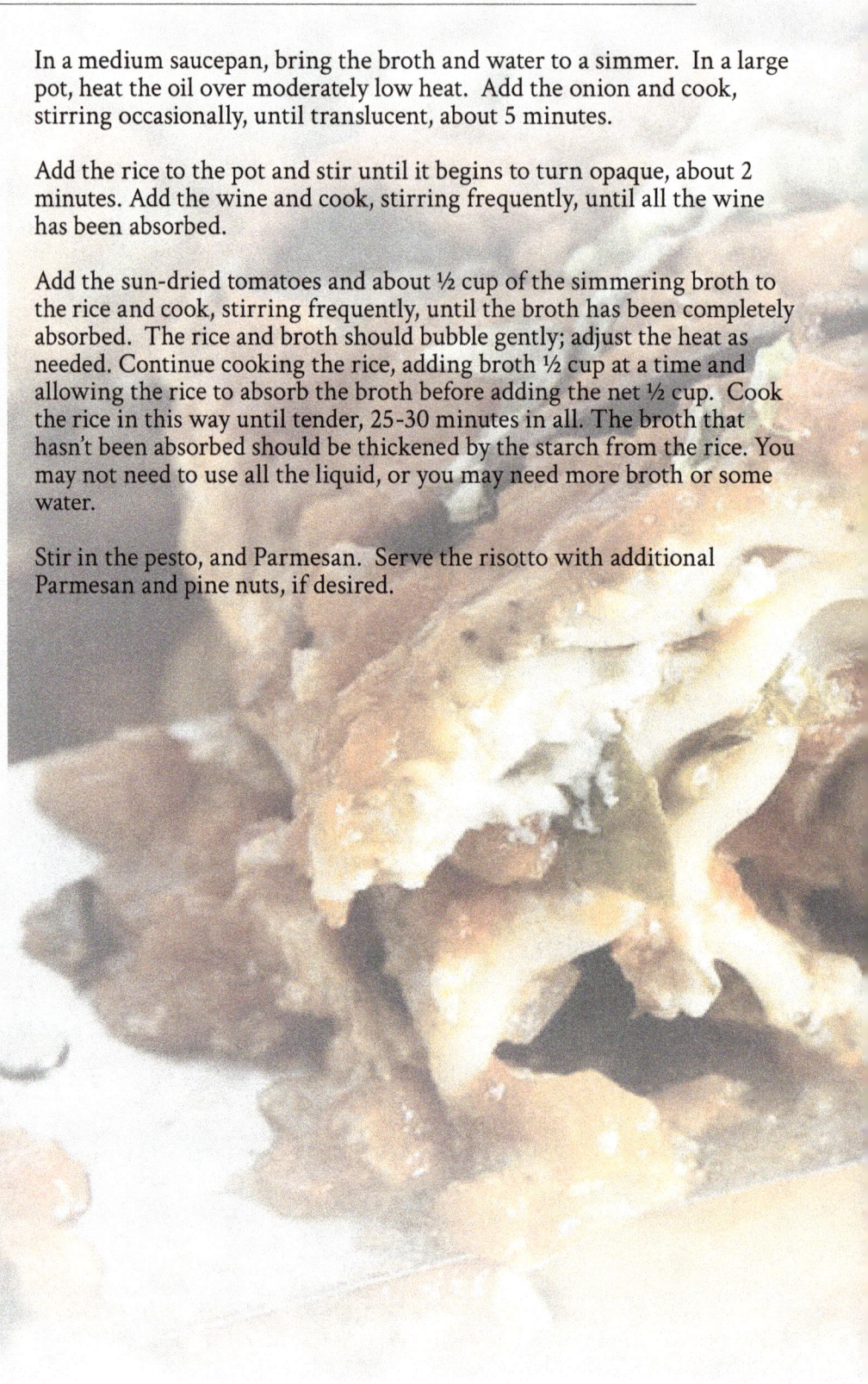

J.R.'s Healthy Lasagna

INGREDIENTS

1-16 oz. box whole wheat lasagna noodles

1 tub fat-free cottage cheese

1 package of fat-free mozzarella cheese

3 small cans of no salt tomato sauce

1 red or white onion, chopped *

1 broccoli floret *

1 red pepper *

1 yellow pepper*

2 carrots, cut up*

1 zucchini, cut in slices*

1 can or bag of frozen corn

1 lb. boneless, skinless chicken breast or 93% or better lean ground beef or turkey burger

1 can of low-sodium black beans

4 cups fresh spinach

3 Tbsp. garlic, minced

2 Tbsp. extra-virgin olive oil*

Many blends of natural seasonings, such as Italian seasoning, oregano, sage, Mrs. Dash, and pepper.

Cut up all the fresh vegetables and spray lasagna pan with nonstick spray.

Cook noodles as directed and rinse with cold water and let stand.

In pan, cook meat until gone and let stand.

In pan, add olive oil letting it heat. Then add vegetables that have a star by them above and cook for 5 minutes.

Add 2nd tier of vegetables and cook about 3 minutes, until all spinach is wilted. Then remove from heat.

Combine meat with the veggies.

Pour 1 can of no salt tomato sauce on bottom of pan. Add 1 layer of noodles; add half of a tub of cottage cheese, half of the meat and vegetables, and a third of mozzarella cheese. Then add another layer of noodles, one more can of sauce, the last of the cottage cheese, and the last of the meat and vegetables, and 2nd third of mozzarella cheese. Add last layer of noodles and last can of sauce, bake on 375 degrees for 30 minutes and remove from oven. Finally, add last of mozzarella cheese and return to oven for 5 minutes. Then remove from oven and let stand for 1 hour in the refrigerator.

Don't be too focused on counting calories…. Instead, focus on color, freshness, and variety. Try to avoid packaged, processed foods. The fresher the better! Simplifying your food decisions will help you avoid frustration and keep you motivated.

Italian Stuffed Shells

INGREDIENTS

24 jumbo whole wheat pasta shells

1 tsp. extra-virgin olive oil

8 oz. can sliced mushrooms

1 can no salt added diced tomatoes

1 can artichoke hearts, drained and coarsely chopped

10 oz. fresh spinach

1 ½ cup fat-free cottage cheese

2 carrots, shredded

1 tsp. dried thyme

½ cup fat-free mozzarella cheese, shredded

Preheat oven to 400 degrees. Prepare pasta per package directions (reducing cooking time by 2 to 3 minute).

Heat oil in large nonstick skillet over medium-high heat. Add mushrooms. Cover and cook, stirring occasionally for about 5 minutes. Add tomatoes (with juice) and artichokes. Cover and simmer for 4 minutes.

Combine remaining ingredients except mozzarella in large bowl. Fill shells with mixture and divide among 8 individual baking dishes coated with cooking spray. Spoon desired amount of sauce over each. Cover loosely with foil and bake 20 minutes. Sprinkle with cheese and bake uncovered 10 minutes or until bubbly.

SERVES

8

Stuffed Shells

INGREDIENTS

18 dry 100% whole wheat jumbo pasta shells

10 oz. fresh spinach, chopped

8 oz. fat-free cottage cheese

½ cup low-fat ricotta cheese

1 cup shredded fat-free mozzarella cheese

2 ½ Tbsp. fresh basil, chopped

2 tsp. oregano

½ tsp. rosemary

2 cups low sodium marinara sauce, divided

Olive oil cooking spray

Cook pasta shells according to package directions, drain and set aside, adding a few drops of oil to prevent sticking. Preheat oven to 350 degrees and lightly coat a roasting pan with cooking spray.

In a large mixing bowl, thoroughly combine spinach, cottage cheese, ricotta, mozzarella, and seasonings.

Pour 1 cup marinara sauce into prepared pan.

Stuff each shell with a heaping tablespoon of filling and place in pan. Pour remaining sauce on top and bake 30 minutes.

SERVES

6

Turkey Pasta Roll-Ups

INGREDIENTS

1 tsp. extra-virgin olive oil

1 Vidalia onion, finely chopped

½ tsp. garlic, minced

1 lb. extra-lean ground white turkey breast

1 tsp. cinnamon

¼ tsp. nutmeg

Any Mrs. Dash seasonings

1-28 oz. can no salt added whole tomatoes in juice

8 sheets dried high-protein or 100% whole wheat lasagna noodles

10 oz. box spinach, chopped

15 oz. container reduced-fat ricotta cheese

1 egg

¾ cup shredded fat-free mozzarella cheese

In a large skillet, heat olive oil over medium heat. Add onion and cook until softened, about 5 minutes. Add garlic and cook another minute. Turn heat to medium-high and add ground turkey, breaking it up with a spatula. Cook until meat shows no sign of pink. Stir in cinnamon, nutmeg, and Mrs. Dash seasonings, then add tomatoes, and their juice. Reduce heat to medium-low, stir, cover, and let simmer for 20 minutes, occasionally stirring and breaking up tomatoes with a wooden spoon.

Meanwhile, bring a large pot of water to boil. Cook pasta according to package directions. Drain, rinse, and allow cooling in a colander.

Preheat oven to 400 degrees. Squeeze all remaining moisture from thawed spinach and place in a large bowl. Add ricotta cheese, egg, and ¼ cup mozzarella cheese to bowl. Stir until combined.

Spread 1 cup of cooked tomato sauce into bottom of a 9" x 10" casserole dish. Lay a cooked lasagna noodle flat in front of you. Use your fingers to spread 1/8 of ricotta mixture across the noodle and roll it up. Place rolled pasta, seam side down, into the casserole dish. Repeat with remaining noodles. Spread remaining tomato sauce over roll-ups, then top with remaining ½ cup mozzarella.

Bake, covered with foil, for 20 minutes. Remove foil and broil for 5 minutes or until roll-ups are browned and bubbly.

SERVES

8

Irish Ravioli

INGREDIENTS

¼ cup firmly packed spinach, chopped

½ cup cannellini (white kidney) beans

½ cup reduced-fat ricotta cheese

2 Tbsp. shredded fat-free mozzarella cheese

32 square wonton wrappers

1 cup unsalted tomato sauce

1 tsp. garlic, minced

Fill a medium saucepan with hot water, cover, and bring to a boil.

While water is heating, defrost the frozen spinach in a microwave. Once thawed, squeeze as much water as you can out of the spinach and place spinach in the bowl of a food processor. Add the beans, cheese, and garlic. Process the bean and cheese mixture until smooth, approximately 1 minute. You should have approximately ¾ cup of ravioli filling.

Fill a small bowl with warm water. Lay out 16 wonton wrappers. Dip you finger in the water and moisten the edges of each wrapper. Place 1 teaspoon of bean-and-cheese filling in the center of each square. From the remaining 16 wrappers, take another wrapper, place it on top of the filling, and seal by pressing firmly along the edges of ravioli. Repeat until all wrappers or filling are used up.

Gently place ravioli in boiling water and cook for approximately two minutes. The ravioli is ready when you can see the green of the filling through the wrappers. While pasta cooks, warm tomato sauce in a small saucepan. Drain pasta and place 4 ravioli on each plate, and top with ¼ cup of sauce.

SERVES

4

Fettuccine

INGREDIENTS

8 oz. 100% whole wheat fettuccine noodles

3 Tbsp. extra-virgin olive oil

1 Tbsp. 100% whole wheat flour

1 can (12 oz.) fat-free evaporated milk

¼ cup green onions, chopped

2 Tbsp. fresh basil, minced

¼ tsp. garlic, minced

¼ tsp. grated lemon peel

1/3 cup grated reduced-fat Parmesan cheese

Additional grated reduced-fat Parmesan cheese and minced fresh basil (optional)

Cook fettuccine according to package directions; drain. Add oil; toss to coat.

In a large saucepan, combine flour and milk until smooth. Stir in the onions, basil, garlic, and lemon peel. Bring to a boil; cook and stir for 2 minutes or until slightly thickened. Remove from the heat; stir in cheese until blended. Pour over fettuccine and toss to coat. Sprinkle with additional cheese and basil if desired.

Muscle Man's Beefy Pasta

INGREDIENTS

1 jar (12 oz.) roasted sweet red peppers, drained

1 lb. lean ground beef

1 white onion, chopped

1 can (14.5 oz.) diced tomatoes, do not drain

1 tsp. garlic, minced

2 tsp. dried oregano

1 ½ tsp. dried basil

½ tsp. red pepper flakes

8 oz. uncooked whole wheat ziti or small tube pasta

1 ½ cups cut fresh green beans

1 ½ cups shredded fat-free mozzarella cheese

Place peppers in a food processor; cover and process until smooth. In a large skillet, cook beef and onion until meat is no longer pink; drain. Stir in the pepper puree, tomatoes, garlic, oregano, basil, and red pepper flakes. Bring to a boil. Reduce heat; simmer, uncovered, for 15 minutes.

Meanwhile, in a Dutch oven, cook pasta according to package directions, adding green beans during the last 5 minutes of cooking. Cook until pasta and green beans are tender; drain. Return to the pan; stir in meat sauce. Sprinkle with cheese; stir until melted.

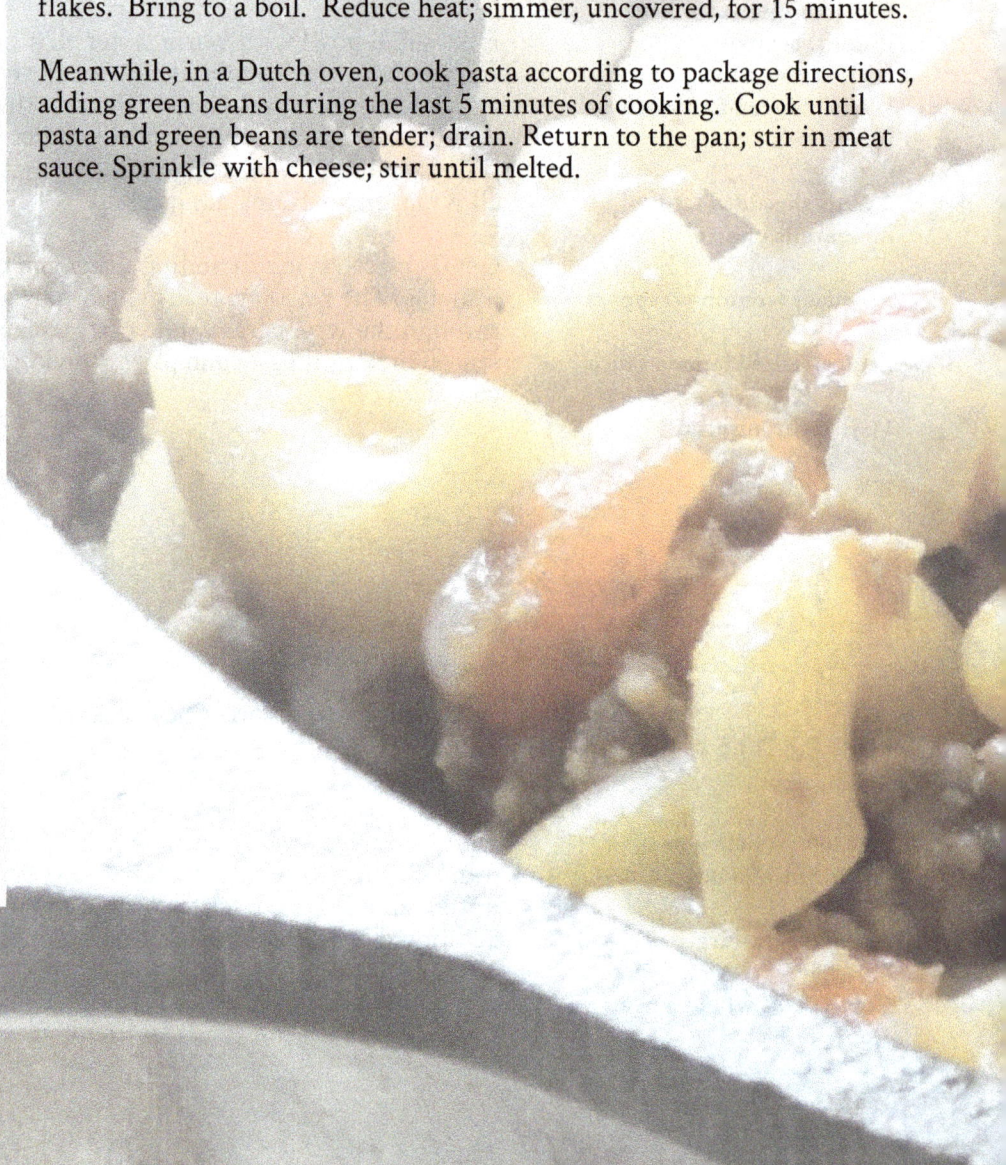

Crabmeat Noodles

INGREDIENTS

8 oz. rice noodles

1 ½ Tbsp. extra-virgin olive oil

1 garlic clove, minced

¼ cup reduced-sodium chicken broth

¼ tsp. red pepper flakes

2 Tbsp. lemon juice

1 Tbsp. capers

8 oz. pasteurized fresh crabmeat

3 Tbsp. chopped parsley

Place rice noodles in a large bowl; fill bowl with hot tap water to soften noodles, approximately 6 minutes.

Meanwhile, heat oil in a large, nonstick skillet over medium heat. Add garlic and cook until slightly golden and fragrant, approximately 1 minute. Add broth and red pepper flakes, and cook for 1 minute. Stir in lemon juice, capers, and crabmeat.

Drain noodles and add to skillet; use tongs to toss and coat noodles with crabmeat mixture, about 1 minute. Remove from heat and garnish with parsley before serving.

SERVES
4

Crab Ravioli

INGREDIENTS

Sauce Ingredients:

1 Tbsp. extra-virgin olive oil

1/3 cup white onion, finely chopped

1 tsp. garlic, minced

28 oz. can crushed tomatoes, do not drain

1 can no salt added diced tomatoes

2 Tbsp. parsley, chopped

1 Tbsp. fresh oregano, chopped

1 tsp. red pepper flakes

½ tsp. black pepper

10 oz. can clams, drained

Ravioli Ingredients:

½ lb. lump crabmeat, drained

½ cup red bell pepper, finely chopped

3 Tbsp. 100% whole wheat panko

1 Tbsp. fresh chives, chopped

½ cup skim milk ricotta

24 round wonton wrappers or gloze skins

To prepare sauce, heat olive oil in a Dutch oven over medium-high heat. Add onion and sauté 3 minutes or until tender. Add garlic and sauté 1 minute. Add crushed and diced tomatoes; bring to a boil. Reduce heat, and simmer 30 minutes. Add the parsley, oregano, red pepper, black pepper, and clams; simmer for 10 minutes. Remove from heat, and set aside.

To prepare ravioli, combine crab, chopped red bell pepper, panko, and chives in a medium bowl. Add ricotta; stir gently to combine. Working with 1 wonton wrapper at a time (cover remaining wrappers with a damp towel to keep them from drying), spoon about 1 Tbsp. crab mixture into center of each wrapper. Moisten edges of wrapper with water. Fold in half, pinching edges together to seal and create a half-moon shape. Repeat procedure with remaining wonton wrappers and crab mixture.

Fill a large Dutch oven with water; bring water to a boil. Add half of ravioli; cook 4 minutes or until done. Remove ravioli from pan with a slotted spoon; keep warm. Repeat procedure with remaining ravioli. Serve ravioli immediately with sauce.

SERVES

6

Scallop Linguine

INGREDIENTS

8 oz. 100% whole wheat linguine

2 Tbsp. extra-virgin olive oil

2 tsp. garlic, chopped

1 Tbsp. shallot, chopped

1-28 oz. can diced tomatoes, drained

½ cup white wine

8 oz. dry sea scallops

¼ cup grated reduced-fat Parmesan cheese

Bring a large pot of water to a boil. Add pasta and cook until just tender, 8 to 10 minutes, or according to package directions. Drain and rinse.

Meanwhile, heat oil in a large skillet over medium heat. Add garlic and shallot and cook, stirring, until beginning to soften, about 1 minute.

Increase the heat to medium-high. Add tomatoes and wine. Bring to a simmer and cook for 1 minute.

Stir in scallops, fish, and marjoram. Cover and cook until the scallops are cooked through and the clams have opened, 3 to 5 minutes more. (Discard any clams that don't open.)

Spoon the sauce over the pasta and sprinkle with additional marjoram and Parmesan.

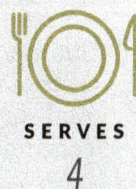

SERVES
4

JR's Shrimp Pasta

INGREDIENTS

1 Tbsp. garlic, minced

½ red onion, chopped

24 oz. medium shrimp, peeled and deveined

1 package imitation crab

1 yellow pepper

1 red pepper

¼ cup parmesan cheese

1 box 100% whole wheat rotini pasta

6 Tbsp. extra-virgin olive oil

Cook box of whole wheat pasta separate.

Cook all other ingredients together and mix with pasta when done. Season with Mrs. Dash spices as desired.

Thai Coconut Shrimp with Brown Rice Pasta

INGREDIENTS

8 oz. brown rice noodles

2 cups broccoli florets

2/3 cup light coconut milk

1 Tbsp. no salt added tomato paste

3 Tbsp. natural peanut butter

2 tsp. ginger, ground

2 tsp. garlic, minced

1 tsp. red pepper flakes

1 Tbsp. lime juice

1 red bell pepper, sliced into thin strips

1 cup bean sprouts

1 cup peapods

24 medium-size raw shrimp or chicken

Bring 2 medium pots of water to a boil over high heat. In 1 pot, cook pasta according to package directions, then rise with hot water to ensure pasta doesn't get sticky when left to stand. (NOTE: Hot water washes away the starch better than cold water when dealing with rice noodles.) Fluff pasta with your fingers or a fork to further de-clump noodles, then set aside. In the second pot of boiling water, add broccoli, cover, turn heat down to low and simmer for 5 minutes. Dain and set aside.

Meanwhile, in a bowl, add coconut milk, tomato paste, peanut butter, ginger, garlic, pepper flakes, and lime juice. Use a fork or whisk to thoroughly combine.

Simmer coconut mixture, bell pepper, and bean sprouts in a nonstick pan over medium-low heat for 5 minutes, stirring often to prevent clumping. Add shrimp and cook for another 2 minutes, then flip shrimp over and continue to cook for a final minute.

Toss noodles, broccoli, and peapods with coconut-shrimp mixture and serve piping hot.

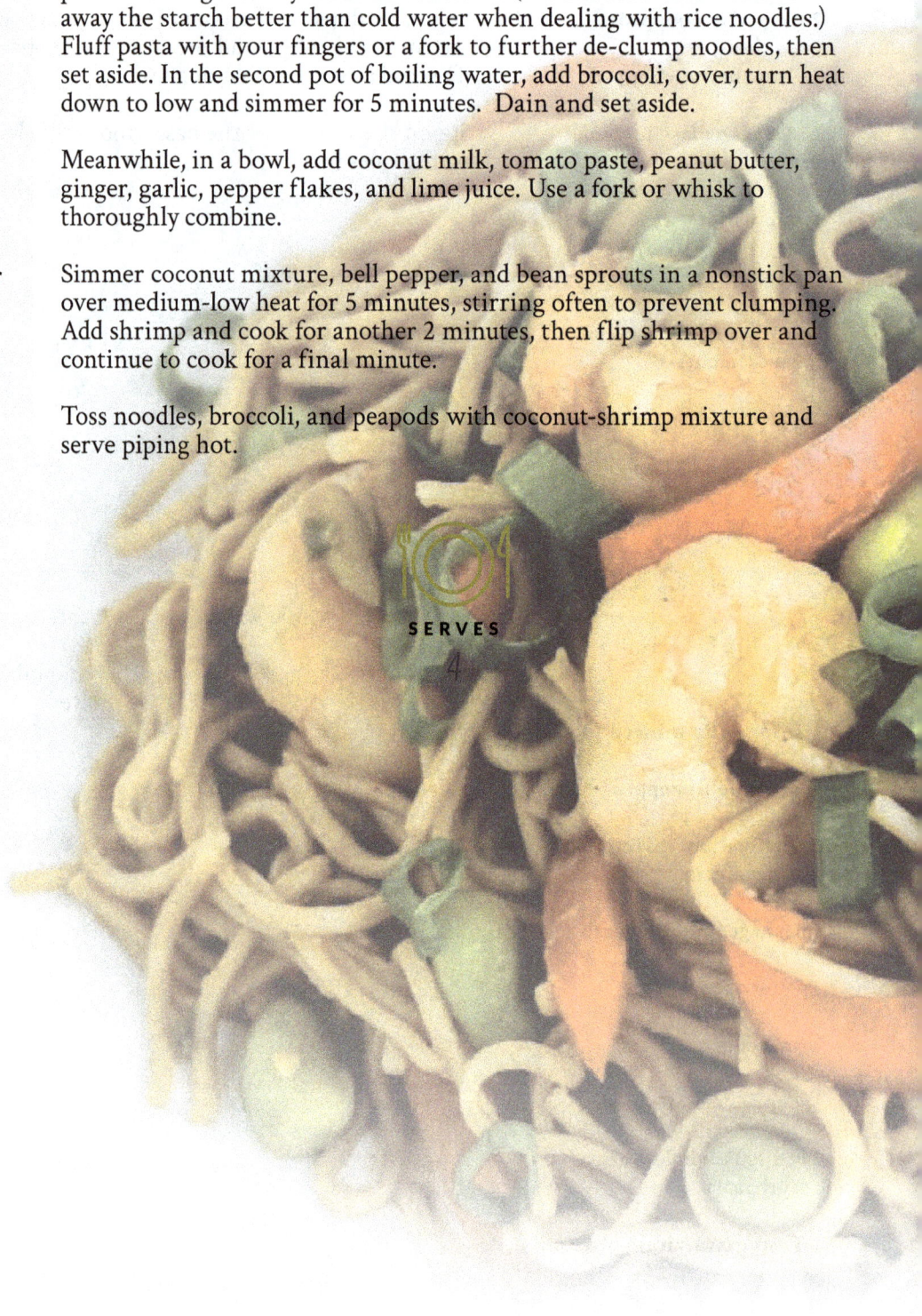

SERVES 4

Shrimp & Edamame Pasta Salad

INGREDIENTS

2 ½ Tbsp. balsamic vinegar

2 Tbsp. Braggs Amino Acid or tamari sauce

1 Tbsp. agave nectar

2 tsp. garlic, minced

12 oz. raw shrimp

8 oz. dried cellophane noodles

1 ½ cups shelled non-frozen edamame

1 Tbsp. refined safflower oil

3 shallots, sliced

¼ cup sunflower sprouts

In a small bowl, combine vinegar, Braggs or tamari sauce, and agave. Set aside.

Fill a large pot with water. Add garlic and bring to a boil over high heat. Remove from heat and add shrimp and noodles. Cover and let stand until shrimp are barely opaque, about 3 minutes. Stir in edamame. Drain, rinse with cold water, and drain again. Remove garlic and set aside.

In a large wok or skillet, heat oil over medium-high heat until it shimmers. Add shallots and stir-fry for 2 minutes, until tender. Remove wok from heat and stir in vinegar mixture. Stir in noodle mixture.

Serve warm or at room temperature, topped with sprouts.

SERVES

4

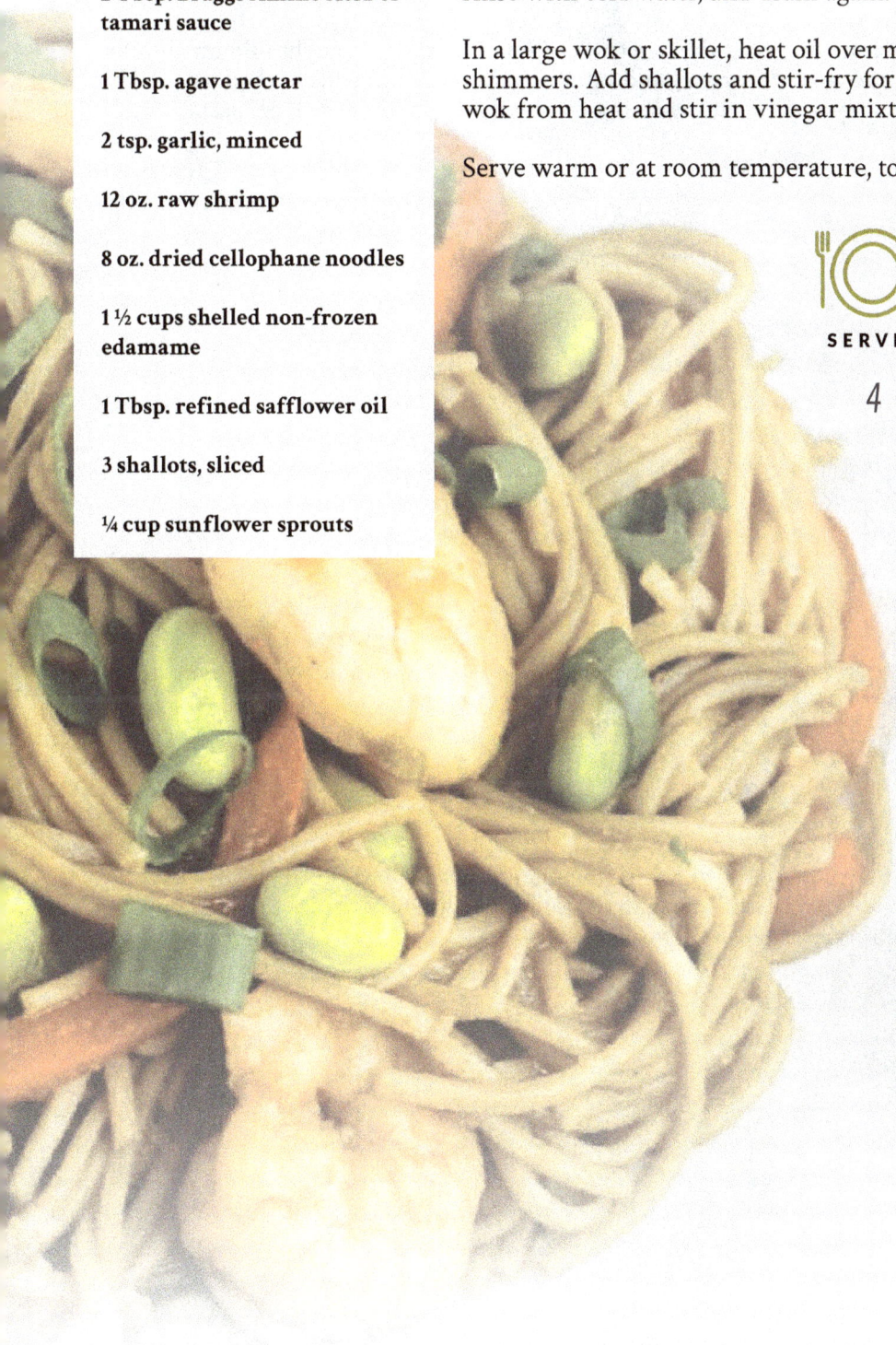

Saffron Salmon Pasta

INGREDIENTS

Sauce Ingredients:

2 cups low-sodium chicken or vegetable broth

1 Tbsp. 100% no sugar added orange juice

4 tsp. arrowroot

½ tsp. saffron threads, crushed

1 Tbsp. extra-virgin olive oil

2 shallots, finely chopped

Pasta Ingredients:

12 oz. wild-caught salmon chunks

Zest of 1-2 oranges

4 cups baby spinach

8 oz. 100% whole wheat linguine

In a medium bowl or measuring cup, whisk together broth, orange juice, arrowroot, and saffron; set aside.

In a medium saucepan over medium heat, warm oil. Add shallots and cook, stirring occasionally, until tender, about 2 minutes.

Stir in broth mixture, increase heat to high and cook, stirring occasionally, until mixture thickens slightly and comes to a boil. Remove from heat and season with salt. Cover and set aside to steep for at least 10 minutes or until ready to serve.

Heat 1½ cups sauce in a skillet. Add 12 oz. wild-caught salmon chunks and zest of 1 orange and simmer, covered, until cooked through. Add 4 cups baby spinach, stirring until wilted. Spoon over 8 oz. pasta.

Clean Ranch Dressing

INGREDIENTS

10 Tbsp. fat-free buttermilk or almond or rice milk

6 Tbsp. fat-free plain Greek yogurt

½ tsp. onion powder

2 tsp. fresh dill, chopped

2 tsp. fresh parsley, chopped

2 tsp. fresh chives, chopped

In a medium bowl, whisk together all ingredients until blended. Refrigerate until serving or use immediately. Store in a sealed container in refrigerator for up to 5 days.

Roman Dressing

INGREDIENTS

4 tomatoes (the type of your choice)

3 Tbsp. apple cider vinegar

2 Tbsp. hemp oil

2 Tbsp. flaxseed oil

6 Tbsp. fresh basil

2 Tbsp. agave nectar

Black pepper and sea salt, to taste

Blend ingredients together.

Ginger Dressing

INGREDIENTS

¾ cup fat-free Greek yogurt

3 Tbsp. Braggs Amino Acid or tamari sauce

6 Tbsp. rice wine vinegar

1 Tbsp. minced garlic

2 Tbsp. Stevia

2 Tbsp. sesame seeds

Mix ingredients all together.

Tzatziki Gyro Sauce

INGREDIENTS

1 cup fat-free plain yogurt

1 cup fat-free plain Greek yogurt

1 ½ Tbsp. lemon juice

1 tsp. cumin

½ tsp. sea salt

1 grated cucumber

Mix ingredients all together.

Pesto Dressing

INGREDIENTS

½ cup pine nuts

1 tsp. clove garlic, peeled

5 cups lightly packed fresh basil leaves

½ cup freshly grated reduced-fat Parmesan cheese

2 Tbsp. fresh lemon juice

¾ cup olive oil

Toast the pine nuts in a small, dry skillet over medium heat until fragrant and golden brown, shaking the pan frequently, about 3 minutes.

In a food processor, process the pine nuts and garlic together until minced. Add the basil, Parmesan, and lemon juice and process until finely minced. With the machine running, slowly pour the oil in a steady stream through the feed tube and process until well blended.

Makes 1 ½ cup, serving size 3 tablespoons

Oriental Dressing

INGREDIENTS

½ cup cold-pressed sesame seed oil

½ cup 100% pure orange juice

¼ cup shallots, finely diced

1 tsp. ginger, finely grated

¼ cup fresh cilantro, finely chopped

¼ tsp. cumin

Add all ingredients to a blender or mini food processor and puree until everything is finely diced.

Summer Curry Salad Dressing

INGREDIENTS

4 Tbsp. white balsamic vinegar

2 Tbsp. apple cider vinegar

1 Tbsp. raw organic honey or Stevia

1 tsp. curry powder

2 tsp. Dijon mustard

Sea salt and fresh ground black pepper, to taste

In a small mixing bowl, whisk together all ingredients. Refrigerate until serving or use immediately.

Store dressing in a sealed container in a cool dark place for up to 6 months.

Herb Dressing

INGREDIENTS

¾ cup fat-free plain Greek yogurt

1 Tbsp. fresh lemon juice

2 tsp. raw organic juice

2 tsp. Dijon mustard

2 tsp. parsley, chopped

2 tsp. fresh dill, snipped or chopped

2 tsp. lemon zest

In a small bowl, whisk together all ingredients until blended. Refrigerate until serving or use immediately. Store in a sealed container in refrigerator for up to 5 days.

Honey Vinaigrette

INGREDIENTS

4 Tbsp. white balsamic vinegar

4 Tbsp. extra-virgin olive oil

2 Tbsp. raw organic honey or Stevia

½ tsp. mustard seeds, ground

Fresh ground black pepper, to taste

In a small mixing bowl, whisk together all ingredients. Refrigerate until serving or use immediately.

Store in a sealed container in refrigerator for up to 2 weeks.

Orange Dressing

INGREDIENTS

4 Tbsp. fresh orange juice

4 Tbsp. white balsamic vinegar or apple cider vinegar

4 Tbsp. extra-virgin olive oil

1 tsp. dried tarragon

½ tsp. dried oregano

1 tsp. orange zest

In a small mixing bowl, whisk together all ingredients. Refrigerate until serving or use immediately.

Store in a sealed container and refrigerate for up to 2 weeks.

Summer Special Vinaigrette

INGREDIENTS

½ cup water

1 cup lemon juice

4 Tbsp. lemon zest

2 Tbsp. organic honey or Stevia

2/3 cup extra-virgin olive oil

2 Tbsp. Dijon mustard

4 Tbsp. dill, chopped

2 Tbsp. shallots, minced

In a blender, blend all ingredients until well mixed. Add salt and pepper to taste.

Brain and emotional health is extremely tied to the foods we eat. Studies have linked eating a typical Western diet-filled with processed meats, packaged meals, takeout food, and sugary snacks-with higher rates of depression, stress, bipolar disorder, and anxiety. If you want to think clearly and support your emotional health, please make wise food decisions.

Homemade Ketchup

INGREDIENTS

3 Tbsp. tomato paste

2 tsp onion powder

2 tsp garlic powder

1 Tbsp. apple cider vinegar

1 tsp raw honey

Combine all ingredients and whisk together. Can be stored in a refrigerator for about a week in a sealed container.

Mexican Dip

INGREDIENTS

1-24oz. container fat free cottage cheese

½ cup fat-free plain Greek yogurt

1 cup bunch scallions

1 cup fat-free or low-fat shredded Mexican 4 Cheese blend

2 tsp. garlic powder

1 tsp. onion powder

2 tsp. garlic, minced

1 tsp. cumin

2 Tbsp. French Onion Dip mix

1 small Jalapeno, seeds removed and chopped

Combine all ingredients and refrigerate for 1 hour.

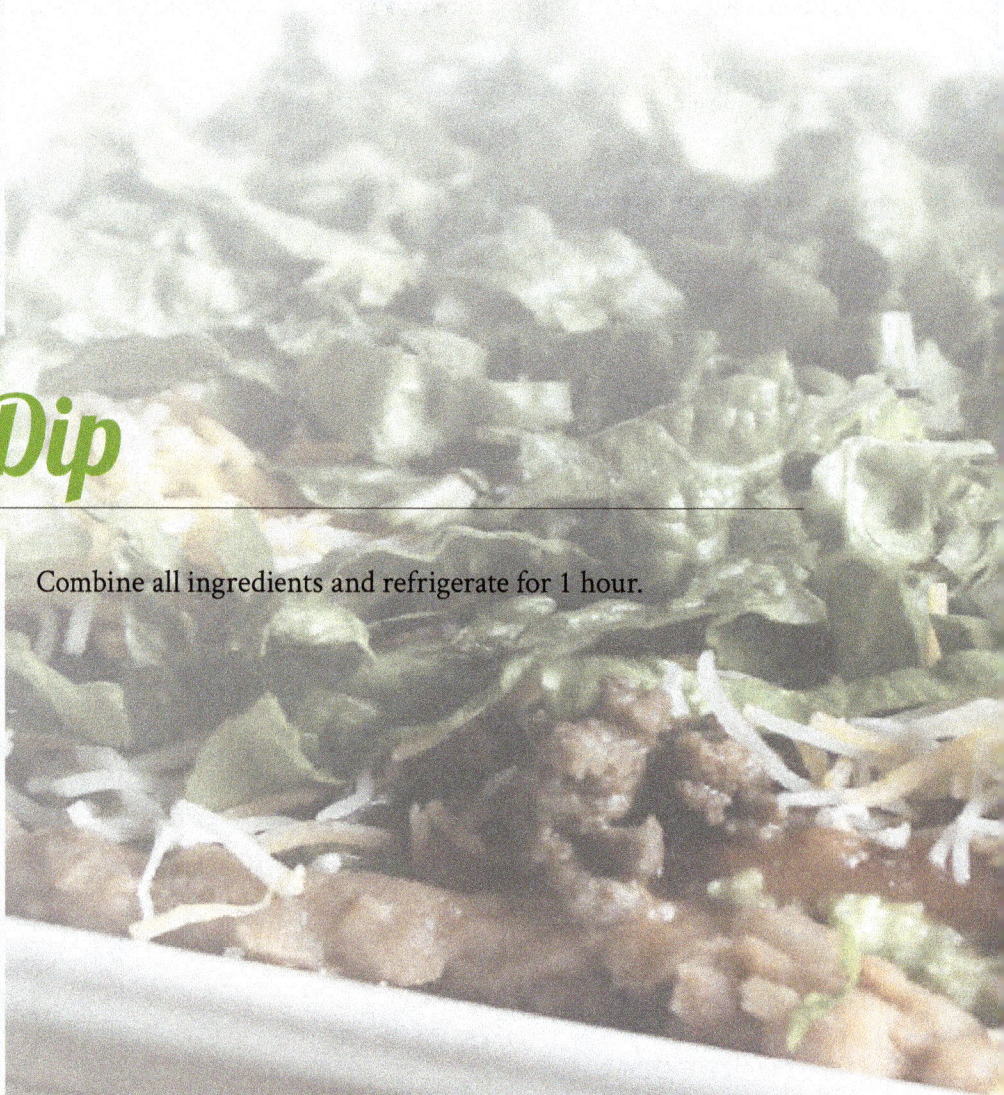

Mexican Party Dip

INGREDIENTS

1 cup dried pinto beans or 1 can of no salt added fat-free pinto/refried beans

2 ½ cups Roma tomatoes, chopped

¾ cup white or red onion, chopped

¼ cup jalapeno peppers, chopped

1 tsp. Tabasco sauce

1 cup packed fresh cilantro leaves, chopped, divided

Juice of 2 limes, divided

2 ripe avocados, pitted and peeled

1 ½ cup fat-free shredded cheddar cheese

1 ½ cups fat-free plain Greek yogurt

Rinse beans in a colander and pick through, discarding any debris or small stones. Place in a medium saucepan and add enough water to cover beans. Bring to a boil over high heat and cook for 2 minutes.

Turn off heat and let beans rest for 1 hour. Drain beans in a colander and rinse. Wash saucepan, return beans to saucepan and add enough water to cover by 2 inches. Bring to a boil over high heat. Reduce heat to low to maintain a steady simmer. Cover and cook for 1 ½ to 2 hours or until beans are very tender. Reserve about 2/3 cup cooking liquid, drain beans and set aside to cook. (Or, cover and refrigerate beans in their cooking liquid for up to 4 days. Reserve 2/3 cup liquid and drain before proceeding with recipe.)

In a medium bowl, combine tomatoes, onion, jalapenos, and about two-thirds of cilantro. Squeeze juice of 1 lime over tomato mixture. Set aside.

In a food processor or blender, combine avocados, remaining cilantro, Tabasco sauce, and remaining juice of 1 lime. Puree until slightly chunky. Set aside.

Place beans and 1/3 cup reserved cooking liquid in a food processor (or use a powerful blender or mash by hand with a potato masher). Process until you have a slightly chunky puree, adding additional cooking liquid, 1 Tbsp. at a time, as needed to reach desired consistency. Pulse several times to combine. Transfer beans to a 9 x 13-inch casserole dish or large glass bowl and spread into an even layer.

Sprinkle cheese evenly over beans. Dollop scoops of avocado mixture over cheese and use a spatula to spread into a thin layer. Dollop scoops of sour cream over avocado and spread into a thick layer. With a slotted spoon (to drain any liquid), spread tomato mixture evenly over sour cream. Serve immediately or cover and chill for up to 4 hours.

Spinach Dip

INGREDIENTS

1 tsp. extra-virgin olive oil

1 cup onion, chopped

2 tsp. garlic, minced

1 pkg. (10 oz.) whole leaf spinach

½ cup fat-free Greek yogurt

1/3 cup almond or rice milk

1 Tbsp. distilled white vinegar

1 tsp. dried dill weed

½ tsp. ground red pepper (cayenne)

1 can water chestnuts, drained and chopped

Dippers: Assorted cut-up raw vegetables and cubed bread

Heat oil in nonstick skillet over medium-high heat. Add onions and garlic and cook, stirring often, until onions are translucent, about 3 minutes. Transfer to a food processor.

Add remaining ingredients, except water chestnuts, and process until almost smooth. Remove processor blade and stir in water chestnuts. Scrape into serving bowl.

Spinach & Ricotta Dip

INGREDIENTS

1 tsp. extra-virgin olive oil

1 ½ Tbsp. garlic, minced

1 leek, washed and thinly sliced

1 ½ cups spinach, coarsely chopped

1 cup reduced-fat ricotta cheese

½ tsp. grated nutmeg

Coat a large, nonstick frying pan with olive oil and set over medium heat. Add garlic and leek. Stir often until soft, 6 to 8 minutes. Add a few drops of water if leek starts to brown too much before it softens.

Increase heat to medium-high heat and add a few handfuls of spinach. Stir until wilted, then turn into a food processor. Continue to cook rest of spinach in small batches until all is wilted. Place in food processor. Whirl until blended—make it as chunky or fine as you like. Turn into a bowl and refrigerate until cool.

Stir spinach with ricotta and nutmeg. Taste and add more seasonings if needed. Dip will water out as it sits; stir before serving.

Red Pepper Hummus

INGREDIENTS

1-15 oz. can garbanzo beans

2 Tbsp. lemon juice

1 Tbsp. garlic, minced

1 Tbsp. sesame seeds

1 Tbsp. extra-virgin olive oil

½ roasted red pepper

1 tsp. ground black pepper

Place all ingredients in food processor and blend until smooth. Serve with vegetables, crackers, or use as a spread.

Loan-Star Caviar

INGREDIENTS

1 cup green, red, and yellow pepper, chopped

1 cup green onion, chopped

1 cup celery, chopped

11 oz. corn, drained

1 small jalapenos, drained and rinsed

1 can pinto beans, drained and rinsed

1 can black beans, drained and rinsed

Any other beans of your choice

Dressing Ingredients:

½ cup Stevia

½ cup cider vinegar

¾ cup extra-virgin olive oil

Mix dressing ingredients in saucepan, bringing to a boil and let cool. Mix remaining ingredients.

Pour dressing over the mixture. Refrigerate overnight.

Drain dressing off before serving.

Black Bean Garden Salsa

INGREDIENTS

1 ¼ cup black beans

2 tomato, diced

2 lime, cut into small pieces

1 onion, diced

2 Tbsp. balsamic vinegar

1 ½ Tbsp. garlic, minced

1 ½ cup cilantro, chopped

1 ½ tsp. dried cayenne pepper

½ Tbsp. hemp oil

½ Tbsp. flaxseed oil

Mix all ingredients together in a bowl. If allowed to sit for a few hours, the ingredients will infuse each other with flavor for an even more delicious mixture

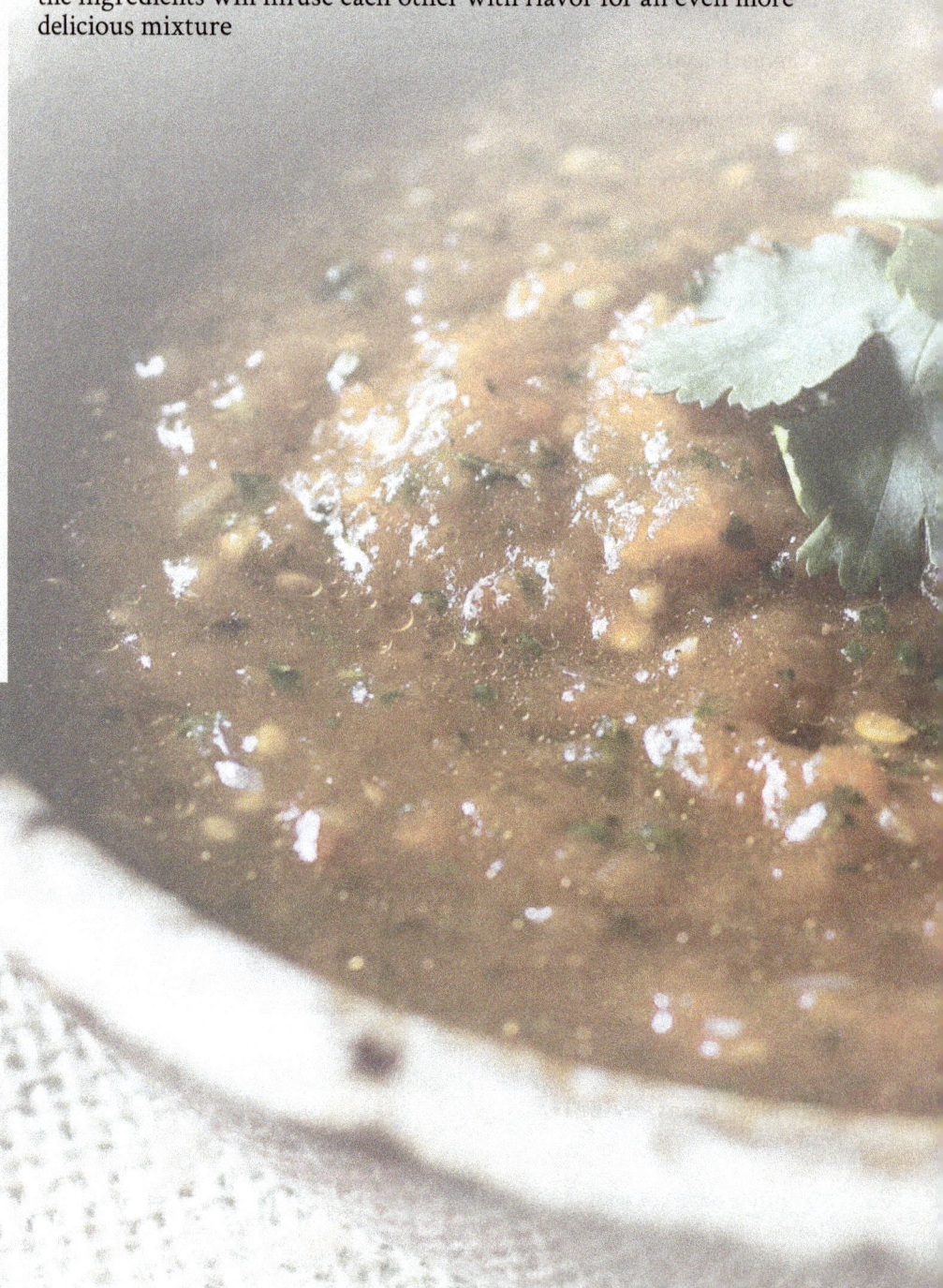

Chipotle Salsa

INGREDIENTS

1 cup corn

½ cup red bell pepper, minced

1 chipotle pepper

1 large red onion, diced, divided

½ tsp. paprika

1 tsp. chili powder, plus additional for garnish

1 Tbsp. extra-virgin olive oil

1 large tomato, chopped

½ tsp. garlic, minced

1 cup black beans, drained and rinsed well

Juice ½ lemon

1 cup cilantro, chopped, divided

In a bowl, combine corn, pepper, half of onion, paprika, and chili powder. Heat oil over medium heat and sauté corn mixture for 5 minutes, stirring occasionally.

In another bowl, combine tomato, garlic, beans, lemon juice, half of cilantro, and remaining half of onion. Toss gently.

Just before serving, toss remaining half of cilantro with corn sauté. Top each salmon (or whatever meat you choose) fillet with ½ cup bean salsa. Then dust corn sauté with additional chili powder and serve alongside salmon and salsa.

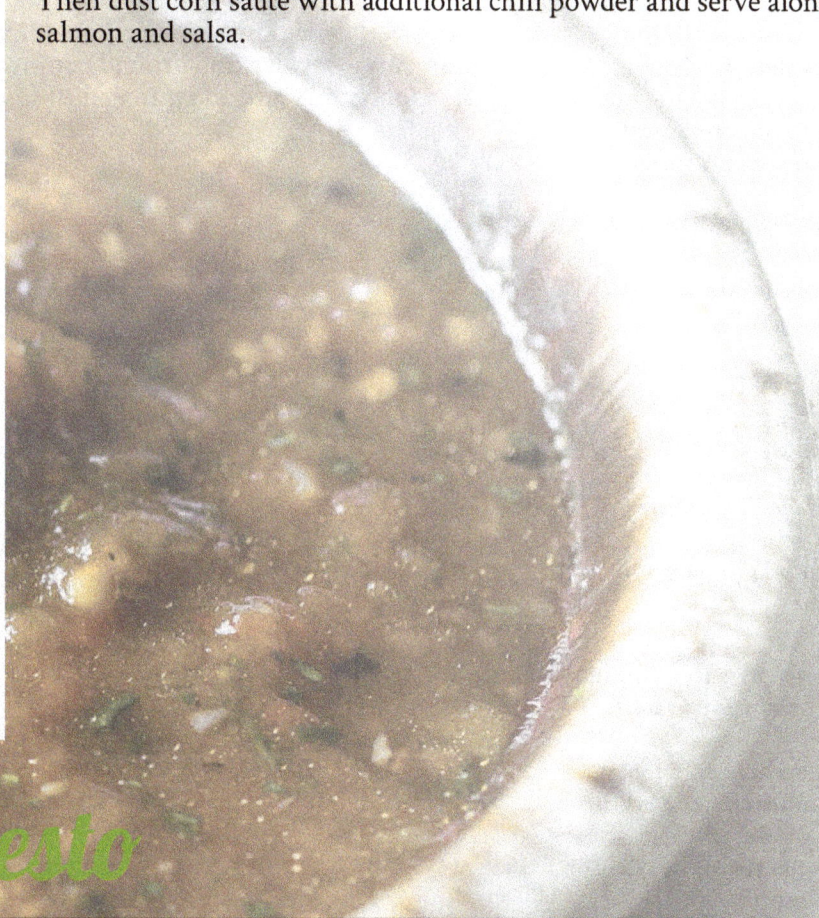

Healthy Pesto

INGREDIENTS

1 bag baby spinach

1 ½ Tbsp. garlic, minced

¼ cup toasted walnuts or pine nuts

1 Tbsp. extra-virgin olive oil

1 cup reduced-fat parmesan cheese

Put all the ingredients in a food processor and mix together. Then use on 100% whole wheat noodles or anything of your choice.

Southern Sweet Potato Pie Spread

INGREDIENTS

2 medium sweet potatoes

1 carrot

1 onion

½ cup water

1 Tbsp. tahini or natural unsalted almond butter

½ tsp. curry powder

1 tsp. ground cumin

In a saucepan, cover sweet potatoes with water and bring to a boil. Simmer over medium heat until potatoes are soft when pierced with a knife (about 30 minutes). Remove from saucepan. When cool, remove skin.

While potatoes are cooking, peel carrot and onion, and chop into small pieces. Place in another saucepan and cover with ½ cup water. Simmer until soft, about 8 minutes.

Puree sweet potato in a food processor along with tahini or almond butter, curry powder, and ground cumin until just combined. Add carrot-onion mixture and puree until smooth.

Peanut Sauce

INGREDIENTS

½ cup creamy natural peanut butter or sunflower butter

¼ cup certified organic, low-sodium chicken broth

3 Tbsp. Braggs Amino Acid or tamari sauce

1 ½ Tbsp. packed dark brown or Sucanat sugar

1 ½ Tbsp. fresh ginger, peeled and minced

2 Tbsp. fresh lime juice

2 tsp. clove garlic, minced

1 tsp. red pepper flakes

1 ½ tsp. red curry paste or curry powder

1 medium shallot, roughly chopped

Place all the ingredients in a blender and blend until smooth. It will keep in the refrigerator for 3 days.

Zucchini Fries

INGREDIENTS

Olive oil cooking spray

4 small zucchini, trimmed and cut into "fries"

½ tsp. sea salt

Freshly ground black pepper, to taste

1 tsp. garlic, minced

1 Tbsp. extra-virgin olive oil

2 Tbsp. reduced-fat, low-sodium Parmigiano-Reggiano cheese, finely grated

Preheat oven to 450 degrees. Line a rimmed baking sheet with foil and coat with cooking spray.

In a large bowl, combine zucchini, salt, pepper, garlic, and oil. Toss to coat thoroughly.

Arrange zucchini on prepared baking sheet in a single layer and roast, tossing once halfway through cooking, for 18 to 20 minutes or until tender and lightly browned. Transfer to a plate, sprinkle with Parmigiano-Reggiano and serve.

SERVES
4

Stuffed Zucchini

INGREDIENTS

3 tsp olive oil, divided

1 clove garlic, minced

½ onion, chopped

3 Tbsp. whole-wheat bread crumbs

2 Tbsp. Parmesan cheese

2 zucchini, halved (seeds and pulp removed)

Heat oven to 350°F.

In large skillet on medium heat, sauté 1 tsp olive oil, garlic, and onion for about 5 minutes. Remove from heat. Add 2 tsp olive oil, bread crumbs, and Parmesan and mix thoroughly. Spoon even amount of stuffing into the zucchini halves.

Bake on foil-lined cookie sheet for about 10 minutes.

Summer Vegetables Medley

INGREDIENTS

1 medium each red and orange bell pepper, stem and seeds removed, sliced into ½-inch strips

1 small green zucchini, cut in half through middle and sliced into ¼-inch strips

1 small yellow zucchini, cut in half through middle and sliced into ¼-inch strips

2 corn ears, husks removed, sliced through core

½ medium white onion, sliced into strips

1 cup dried navy beans, soaked overnight and boiled or 1 can black beans

1 ½ tsp. dried Herbs de Provence blend

1 Tbsp. garlic, minced

2 Tbsp. white balsamic vinegar

1 Tbsp. extra-virgin olive oil

1 tsp. ground black pepper

2 tsp. parsley

4 oz. goat cheese, crumbled or fat-free herb feta cheese

Preheat oven to 350 degrees.

In a large mixing bowl, add bell peppers, zucchini, corn, and onion.

Add beans, Herbs de Provence, garlic, vinegar, and oil to vegetables. Toss to combine and season with black pepper and parsley.

Prepare 3 foil pouches, dividing vegetable mixture evenly among foil pouches and seal. Place pouches on a baking tray and slide onto middle rack of preheated oven. Roast for 25 minutes or until vegetables have softened slightly. Remove pouches from oven and carefully open to rest for doneness. (Vegetables should be soft and still a bit crunchy.)

To serve, divide vegetables evenly among 4 plates. Top each serving with 1 oz. cheese, if desired.

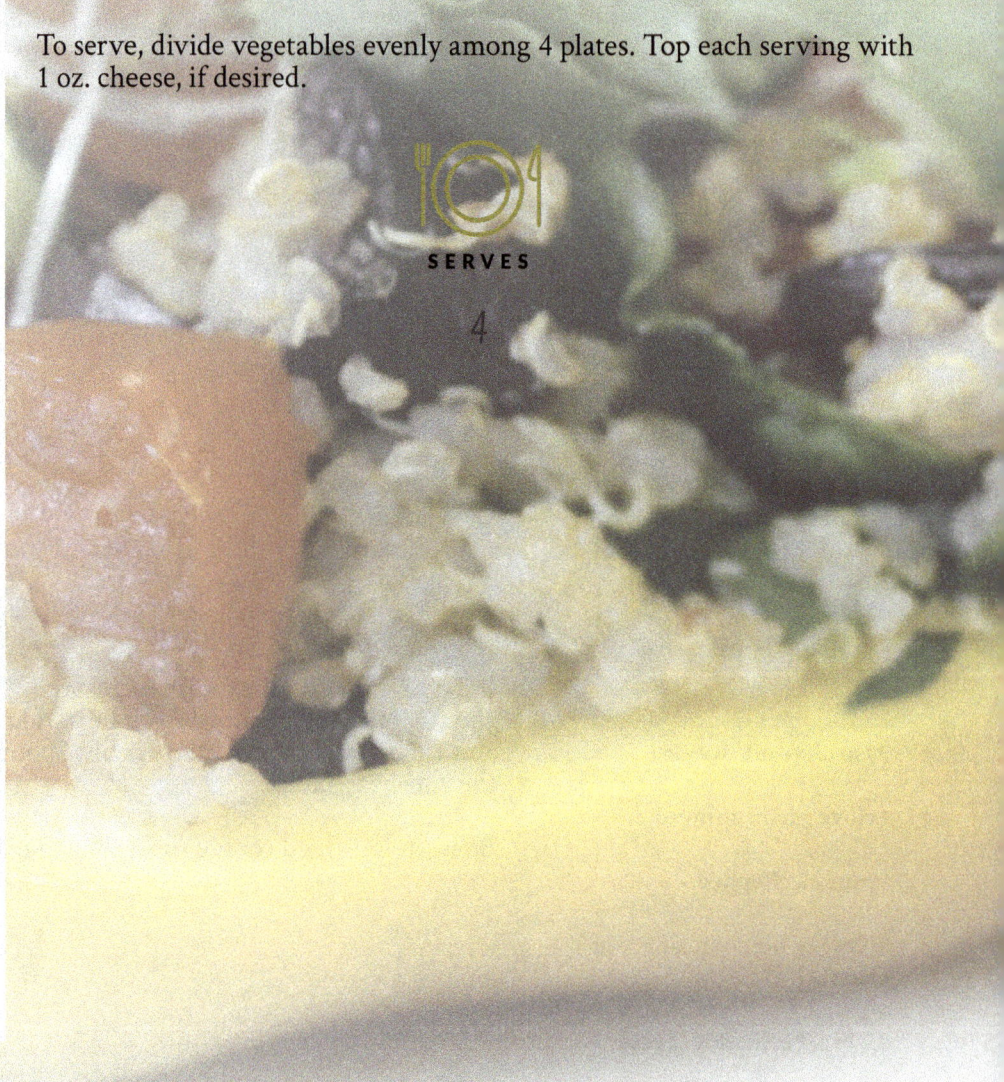

SERVES

4

Gluten-Free Stuffed Power Peppers

INGREDIENTS

4 peppers, colors of your choice

3 cups cooked quinoa

1 cup fat-free cottage cheese

2 boneless, skinless chicken breasts, cooked and shredded

1 can no salt added tomatoes, drained

Preheat oven to 350 degrees. Cut peppers in half and remove stems and seeds.

Mix chicken, quinoa, cottage cheese, and tomatoes. Stuff peppers and place in sprayed baking dish with ¼ cup water in bottom of pan. Cover with foil.

Cook for 45-60 minutes or until peppers are tender.

SERVES
4

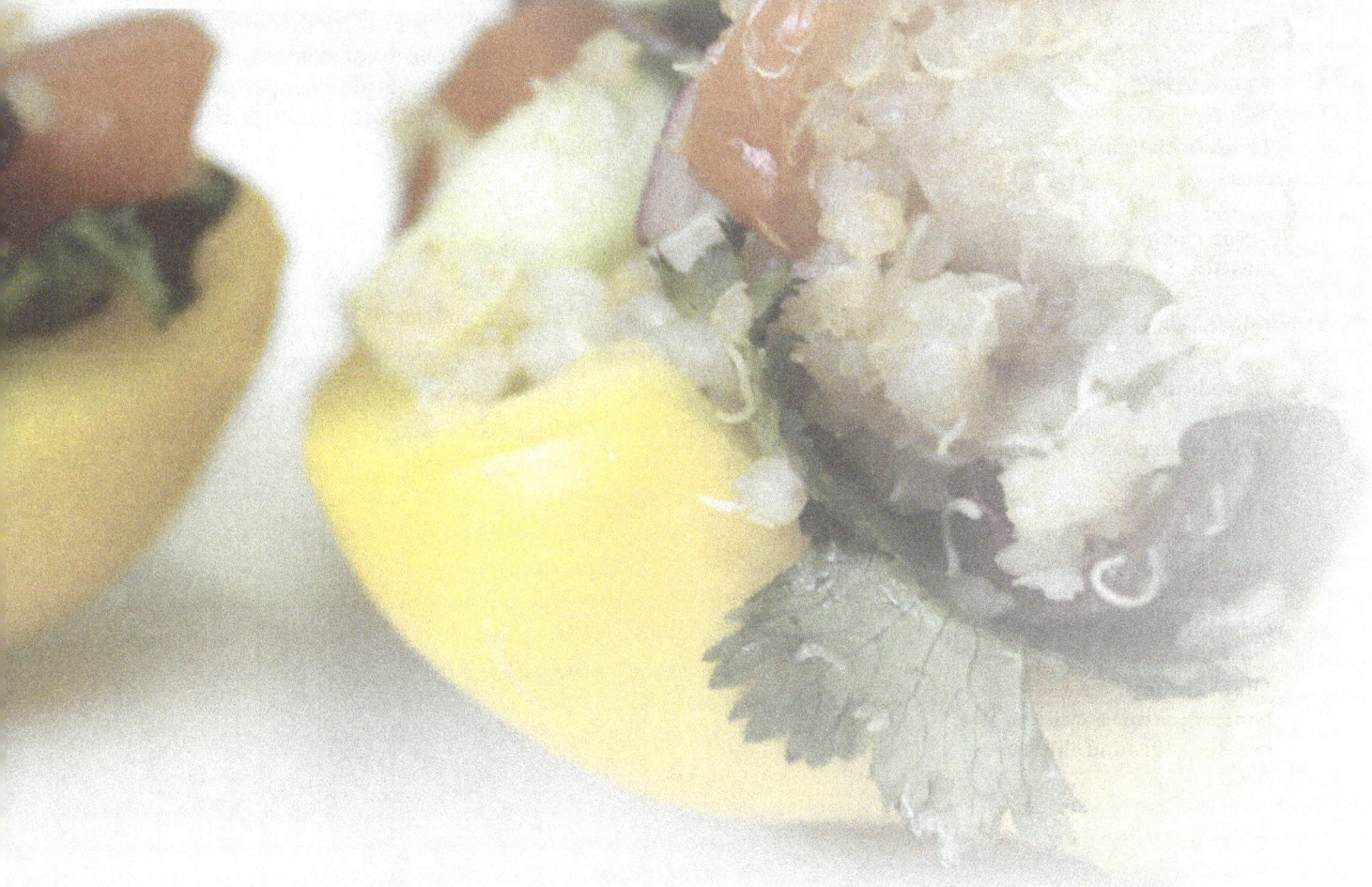

Mexican Stuffed Peppers

INGREDIENTS

4 large red bell peppers (or any color of your choice)—make sure the peppers are able to sit upright without fall over.

2 cups brown rice

1 tsp. extra-virgin olive oil

1 red onion, chopped

1 large carrot, grated

1 cup butternut squash, peeled and diced

2 Tbsp. garlic, minced

2 cups fresh Roma tomatoes, diced

1-15 oz. can black beans, rinsed and drained

1 cup fresh corn kernels

½ zucchini

½ cup fresh cilantro, chopped

2 Tbsp. fresh lime juice

½ tsp. ground black pepper

Olive oil cooking spray

1 lb. of any lean meat—boneless, skinless chicken breasts, or ground chicken or turkey

Preheat oven to 350 degrees. Place cooked brown rice in a bowl and let cool. Set aside.

Make sure there is a rack in the middle of the oven. Bring a large pot of salted water to a boil. Place the peppers in the boiling water and cook briefly. The peppers need to be just a little soft. Remove the peppers from the water and put them on a plate lined with paper towels, upside down so the water can drain out.

In a large skillet, heat olive oil and sauté onion, carrot, and butternut squash. Cook for 10 minutes, covered. Add garlic and cook a few minutes more. Now add tomatoes, beans, corn, and zucchini.

Cook for 5 minutes. Remove from heat.

Add vegetable mixture to cooked brown rice. Season with cilantro, lime juice, and black pepper. Mix with clean, bare hands until all ingredients are evenly distributed. Set aside.

Prepare a small baking pan with a light coating of nonstick spray. Place each of the peppers right-side up in the pan. Stuff each pepper with brown rice filling. Don't pack the rice mixture too tightly. Bake for 20 minutes. Remove from heat and serve immediately.

If you have left over filling, it tastes delicious in a 100% whole wheat tortilla

SERVES

4

Spaghetti Squash Salad

INGREDIENTS

3 Tbsp. red wine vinegar

2 tsp. extra-virgin olive oil

2 tsp. dried oregano

¼ tsp. black pepper

2 garlic cloves, minced

3 cups cooked spaghetti squash

2 cups tomato, chopped

1 ½ cup cucumber, diced

½ cup (2 ounces) crumbled fat-free feta cheese

½ cup green bell pepper, diced

¼ cup red onion, diced

2 Tbsp. pitted kalamata olives

1 (15 ½ ounce) can chickpeas (garbanzo beans), drained

Combine first 6 ingredients into a bowl; stir well with a whisk.

Combine squash and remaining ingredients in a large bowl. Add vinegar mixture; toss well. Cover and chill.

SERVES

8

Eggplant Parmigiana

INGREDIENTS

1 large eggplant, sliced

1 1/2 cups kale, minced

1/3 cup whole wheat flour

1 cup egg whites

½ cup olive oil

1 ½ cups marinara (homemade)

1 tomato, finely diced

1 clove garlic, minced

2 cups mozzarella cheese

½ cup parmesan cheese

Ground pepper to taste

Preheat oven to 375°

Use two small bowls, one for flour and the other for egg whites. Lightly coat eggplant with flour by dipping into bowl, then dip into egg whites. Place coated eggplant in large skillet on medium heat with olive oil. Sauté for about 10 minutes (5 minutes on each side). Continue until all slices are sautéed.

In baking dish, add ½ cup of marinara to the bottom. Add in layers in order: the sautéed eggplant, minced kale, diced tomato, and mozzarella. Repeat layers with remaining ingredients. Add the remaining marinara to the top. Then, add the parmesan cheese and ground pepper to the top. Bake for about 20 minutes.

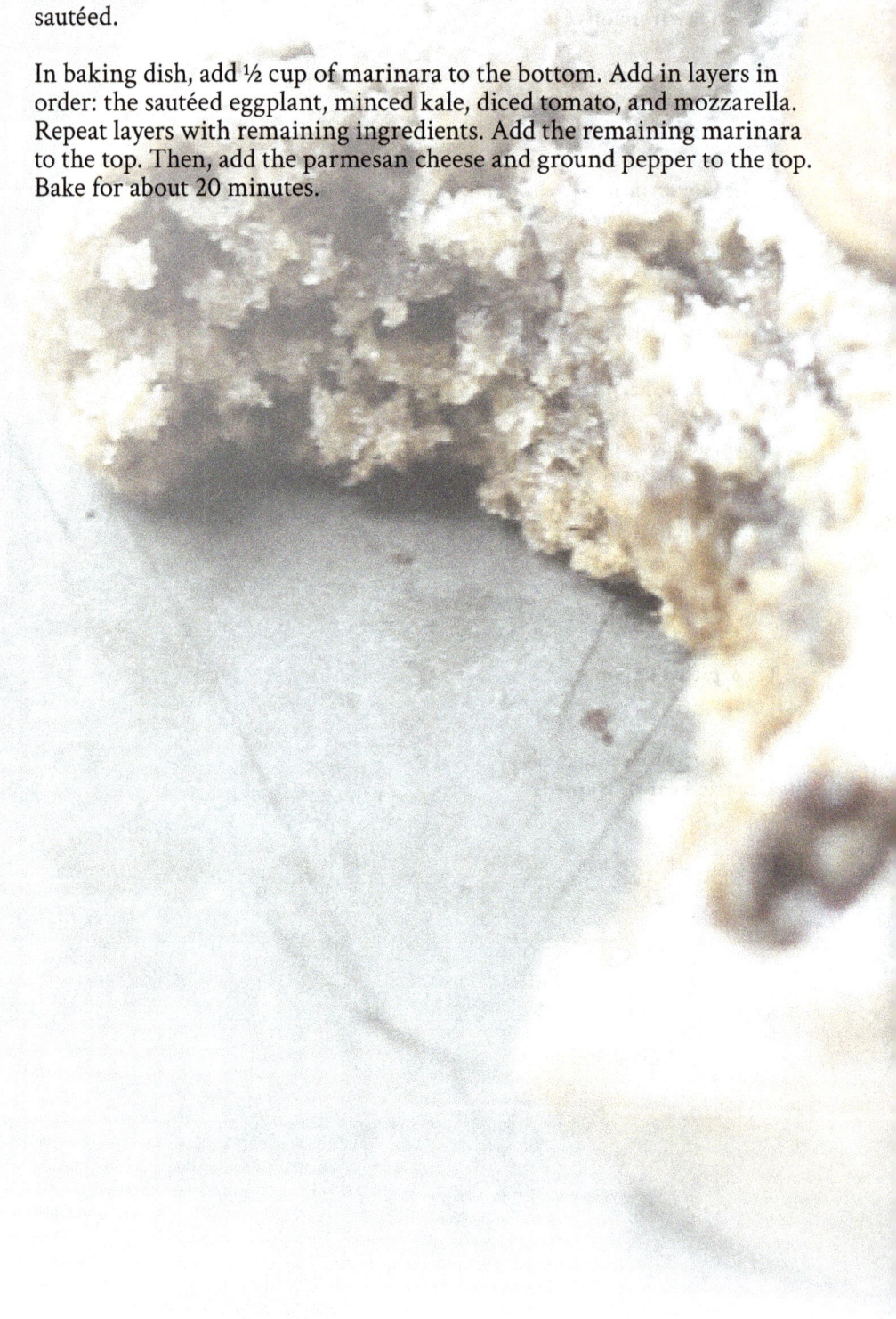

Power Cookies

INGREDIENTS

1 ½ cups 100% whole wheat flour

2 cups whey protein powder (vanilla tastes best)

1 tsp. baking powder

1 Tbsp. cinnamon

1 ½ cups fat-free cottage cheese

½ cup honey or agave nectar

¼ cup extra-virgin olive oil

1 egg

2 tsp. vanilla extract

1 cup rolled oats

½ cup semisweet chocolate chips

½ cup walnuts, chopped

Preheat oven to 350 degrees.

Combine first 4 ingredients in a large bowl and blend with a fork.

In a separate bowl, combine next 5 ingredients and whisk together with a fork, or use an electric mixer or food processor.

Add wet ingredients to dry and mix with a fork. Mix in oats, chocolate chips, and walnuts.

Drop by the teaspoonful onto an oiled or parchment-paper-lined baking sheet. Bake 12 minutes until the cookies are slightly brown on top.

SERVES
30

Chocolate Almond Butter Gluten Free Cookies

INGREDIENTS

1 cup unsalted almond butter, stirred well

¾ cup Sucanat

1 large egg

½ tsp. baking soda

1 tsp. cinnamon

3 oz. dark chocolate (70% cocoa or greater), broken into small pieces

Preheat oven to 350 degrees. In a medium bowl, stir together first 5 ingredients until blended. Stir in chocolate.

Drop dough by rounded the tablespoonful onto parchment-lined baking sheets. Bake for 10 to 12 minutes or until lightly browned. Let cool on baking sheets for 5 minutes. Remove to a wire rack and let cool for 15 more minutes.

SERVES
24

Guilt Free Brownies

INGREDIENTS

1 can low-sodium black beans, rinsed and drained

3 whole eggs

2 tsp. vanilla extract

12 oz. package extra-firm lit tofu

½ cup unsweetened applesauce

2 Tbsp. olive oil

1/3 cup pure maple syrup or agave nectar

½ cup unsweetened, non-dutched (unprocessed) cocoa

¾ cup chocolate whey protein powder

1 tsp. baking powder

1 Tbsp. cinnamon

Preheat oven to 350 degrees.

Puree beans in a food processor. Add the rest of the wet ingredients and blend to combine.

In a large mixing bowl, use a fork to mix together the dry ingredients. Add to the wet ingredients and blend until creamy smooth.

Pour batter into an oiled 8-by-8-inch baking dish. Bake for 30 minutes or until a knife inserted in the center comes out clean.

SERVES

16

Nutty Chocolate Squares

INGREDIENTS

½ cup unsalted raw walnuts or hazelnuts, coarsely chopped

1 ½ cups unsweetened brown rice cereal

¾ cup rolled oats

3 tsp. cinnamon

2 ½ oz. (1/3 cup + 2 Tbsp..) dark chocolate (70% cocoa or greater), chopped into chunks

1 cup unsweetened dried pitted dates, pureed until smooth.

½ cup unsalted hazelnut butter or your favorite unsalted natural nut butter

2 Tbsp. raw honey, Stevia, or agave nectar

In a medium mixing bowl, add hazelnuts, cereal, oats, and cinnamon and stir until combined. Set aside.

Melt chocolate in a medium bowl over a double boiler. Remove bowl from double boiler and, using a wooden spoon, add pureed dates, hazelnut butter, and honey, Stevia, or agave nectar to melted chocolate. Carefully stir until combined. As mixture stiffens, set bowl over double boiler again as needed.

Add chocolate mixture to bowl with cereal mixture and fold in until thoroughly combined. Scrape mixture into baking pan (9 x 11 x 2 inches), pressing down firmly with your hands and smoothing the top. Cover and refrigerate for 30 minutes to 1 hour to allow mixture to set. Cut into 1 ½-inch squares and serve immediately. Squares can be kept, covered, in refrigerator for 3 to 5 days.

***Try serving squares with a bit of strained fat-free plain yogurt sweetened with raw honey.

***Instead of using a baking pan, you can also roll your chocolate-cereal mixture into truffle-like balls before refrigerating (1 ½ Tbsp. mixture each; makes about 24 balls)

SERVES

24

Cheesecake Pears

INGREDIENTS

10 pears

2 cinnamon sticks

2 cups each 100% cranberry juice and 100% orange juice

1 vanilla bean, split lengthwise

Cheesecake Stuffing:

1 cup fat-free cream cheese, at room temperature

2 tsp. vanilla extract

½ tsp. dried ginger

1 Tbsp. cinnamon

1/3 cup dried unsweetened cranberries

½ cup unsalted, sliced almonds, toasted

Peel pears. Trim bottoms so that they sit flat. Using a small spoon or a melon baller, scoop out and discard cores. Place pears in a very large, wide, heavy-bottomed saucepan. Add cinnamon sticks and juices. Scrape out seeds from vanilla bean and stir in; add scraped bean husks, too.

Bring to a boil, then reduce heat. Cover and simmer, occasionally turning pears over carefully to ensure even cooking, until almost tender but still a little firm, about 20 to 25 minutes.

In a bowl, stir cream cheese with vanilla extract, ginger, and cinnamon until mixed. If the mixture is too thick to stir easily, add a few spoonfuls of hot pear cooking liquid. Stir in cranberries and almonds.

Carefully spoon pears onto a large platter. Cover and refrigerate to cook completely. Boil remaining pear liquid in pan, stirring often, until it reduces to ½ cup. The sauce will foam and bubble toward the end of cooking, so be sure to stir often. Remove from heat and discard cinnamon sticks and vanilla husks.

To serve, fill pears with cream cheese mixture. Place on plates and spoon sauce over the top.

***Refrigerate for up to 3 days. Poach pears and make the sauce. Refrigerate overnight. Stuff pears and keep refrigerated for up to 6 hours. Bring both pears and sauce to room temperature before serving.

SERVES

10

Apple-Berry Crumble

INGREDIENTS

1 lb cooking apples

1 Tbsp. lemon juice

1 cup fresh blackberries or unsweetened frozen blackberries, or any other berries

¼ cup 100% whole wheat flour or gluten-free brown rice flour

¼ cup rolled oats

1 tsp. cinnamon

3 Tbsp. extra-virgin olive oil

¼ cup pitted dates, finely chopped

¼ cup unsalted sunflower seeds

Olive oil cooking spray

Preheat oven to 400 degrees. Prepare an ovenproof dish by coating with cooking spray.

Core and slice the unpeeled apples and sprinkle with lemon juice. This helps prevent browning. Place in a medium saucepan with the blackberries. Cook over medium-low heat and bring to a simmer.

Simmer for 5 minutes. Pour cooked fruit into baking dish.

In a separate bowl, mix the flour, oats, and cinnamon. Rub in the oil and stir until mixture resembles crumbs. You may need to add more olive oil until desired texture is reached. Stir in dates and sunflower seeds. Sprinkle crumbly mixture over fruit. Bake in the oven for 25 minutes.

SERVES

4

Apple Crisp

INGREDIENTS

2 Gala apples

2 Tbsp. Stevia

¼ cup old-fashion oats

1 Tbsp. cinnamon

½ tsp. nutmeg

Heat oven to 350 degrees. Arrange apple slices in baking pan, coated with nonfat cooking spray. Mix remaining ingredients sprinkle over apples.

Bake for 30-35 minutes or until topping is golden brown and apples are tender.

SERVES
1

Healthy Fudge Cakes

INGREDIENTS

Olive oil cooking spray

1 oz. dark organic chocolate (70% cocoa or greater)

1 Tbsp. water

1 ½ cups soft-cooked black beans, rinsed and drained

2 eggs

1 egg white

2 Tbsp. extra-virgin olive oil

¼ heaped cup unsweetened cocoa powder

1 tsp. baking powder

1 Tbsp. cinnamon

1 tsp. vanilla extract

¼ cup unsweetened applesauce

½ cup raw organic honey, Stevia, or agave nectar

¼ cup unsalted walnuts, chopped

Preheat oven to 350 degrees. Mist 8 individual ramekins or 1 8-inch square baking dish with cooking spray.

Melt dark chocolate in a small saucepan over low heat with 1 Tbsp. water mixed in.

Combine melted chocolate, beans, eggs, egg white, oil, cocoa powder, baking powder, cinnamon, vanilla, applesauce, and honey, Stevia, or agave nectar in a food processor; process until smooth. Stir in walnuts and pour mixture into prepared ramekins or baking dish.

Bake in preheated oven until the tops are dry and the edges start to pull away from the sides, about 20 minutes for ramekins and 30 minutes for baking dish. Garnish each piece with a dollop of fat-free Greek yogurt, if desired.

SERVES
8

Peanut Butter Fudge Bars

INGREDIENTS

4 scoops chocolate protein powder

2/3 cup flax meal

2 tsp. cinnamon

4 Tbsp. natural peanut butter, unsalted

¼ cup water

1 tsp. Stevia

Mix all ingredients in a large bowl and stir. At first, it may seem like it's not enough water, but keep stirring and it will eventually become a sticky blob of dough. Add 1 Tbsp. water at a time, if needed.

Divide the mixture into 4 equal portions and place in separate pieces of plastic wrap, shaping them into bars. It's easier to shape them by lying plastic wrap on one side of a small casserole dish, pressing the dough into the natural shape of the dish.

Store the bars in the fridge or freezer. You can eat them chilled or frozen.

Bake Free Bars

INGREDIENTS

Olive oil cooking spray

1 ½ cup dry oatmeal

2 scoops chocolate whey protein

2 Tbsp. flaxseeds

1 Tbsp. cinnamon

1 cup fat-free powdered milk

¼ cup all natural peanut butter

¼ cup water

2 tsp. vanilla extract

½ cup raisins or any other unsweetened fruit of your choice

Lightly spray an 8-inch square pan with cooking spray.

In a large bowl mix oatmeal, whey protein, flaxseeds, cinnamon, and powdered milk.

In a separate bowl, whisk together peanut butter, water, and vanilla. Add the peanut butter mixture to the dry ingredients and stir to form sticky dough. Stir or knead in the raisins.

Using wet hands or a spatula, spread the mixture evenly into the prepared 8-inch pan. Freeze for 1 hour (or refrigerate overnight) until mixture is firm enough to cut. Cut into 9 squares. Wrap individually and store in your refrigerator.

SERVES

9

Post-Workout Truffles

INGREDIENTS

1 cup prunes

½ cup warm water

¼ cup natural almond or peanut butter

1 cup protein powder

¼ cup ground flaxseeds

3 Tbsp. sesame seeds

1 tsp. cinnamon

½ cup dried unsweetened cranberries

½ cup wheat germ, divided

Place prunes in warm water for 10 minutes to soften.

In a food processor, blend prunes and water. Add nut butter and process until smooth. Add more water as needed. Add protein powder, flaxseed, sesame seeds, and cinnamon, and process to combine thoroughly. Add the cranberries and ¼ cup wheat germ and pulse just enough to incorporate them into the mixture.

Grab some dough about the size of a small ball and roll between your palms. If dough becomes too sticky, place it in the freezer for 15 minutes. Roll each ball in the wheat germ to coat. Set balls on a baking sheet and place in the freezer when done. Allow the balls to freeze for 2 to 4 hours. Then store in an airtight container either in the freezer or refrigerator.

SERVES

35

The Great Chocolate Pudding

INGREDIENTS

1 pint Greek yogurt

2 scoops chocolate protein powder

2 packets stevia

4 tsp cocoa powder

Combine all ingredients. Top with your favorite fruit or nuts.

The Great Vanilla Pudding

Combine all ingredients. Top with your favorite fruit or nuts.

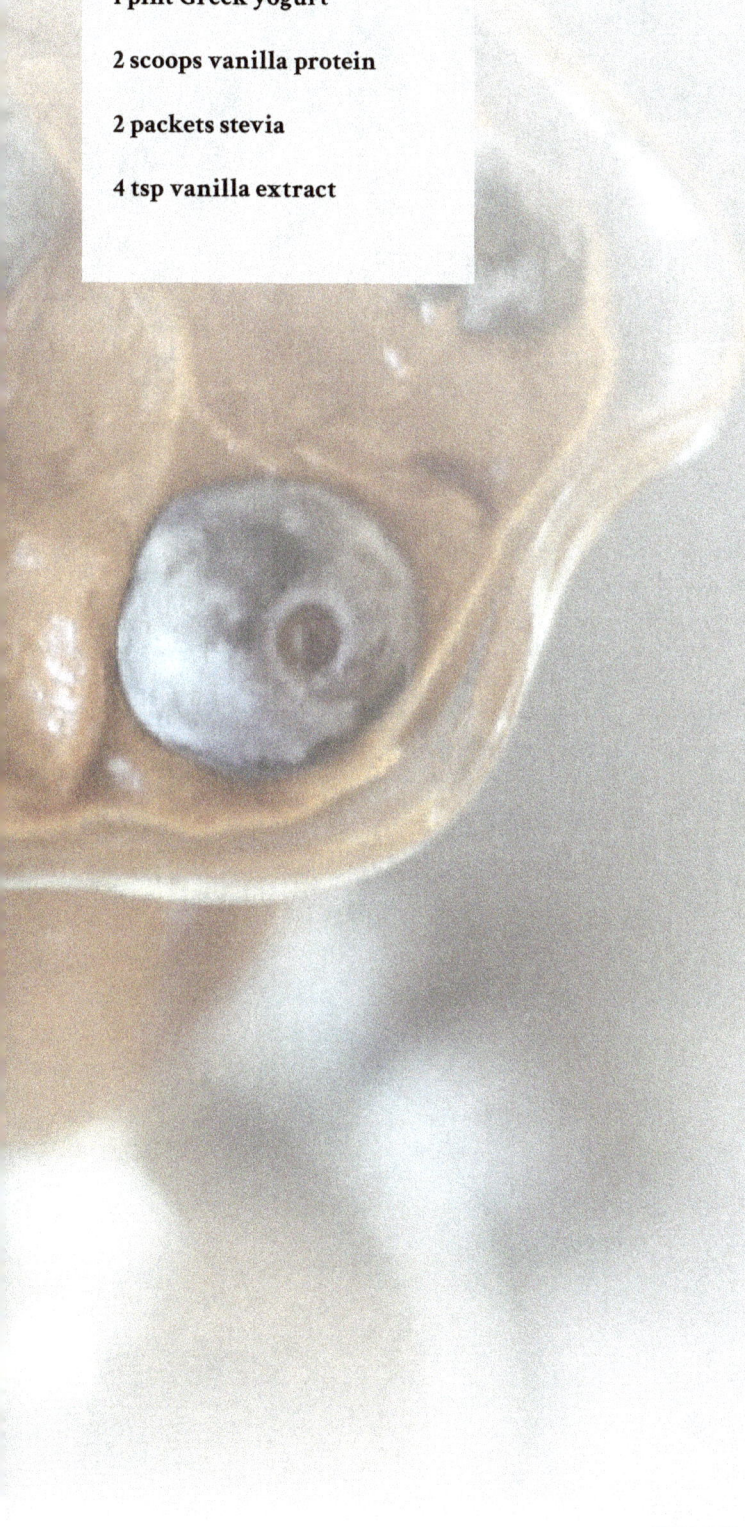

INGREDIENTS

1 pint Greek yogurt

2 scoops vanilla protein

2 packets stevia

4 tsp vanilla extract

PHASE 3

WITH PHASE 3, YOU ENTER THE MAINTENANCE PHASE OF YOUR HEALTH JOURNEY. HERE YOU HAVE REACHED YOUR WEIGHT, CHOLESTEROL, BLOOD SUGAR, OR OTHER HEALTH GOALS AND YOU WANT TO MAINTAIN THAT ACHIEVEMENT. YOU MUST CONTINUE TO USE THE CONTROL AND PRINCIPLES OF LOW GLYCEMIC FOODS, MEAL SIZE, AND FREQUENCY TO MAINTAIN YOUR METABOLISM AND HEALTH. DURING PHASE 3, YOU NEED TO CONTINUE TO MONITOR YOUR WEIGHT AND BODY FAT PERCENTAGES TO KEEP ON TRACK. YOU CAN ADD BACK AN EXTRA SERVING OF WHOLE GRAIN BUT CONTINUE TO HAVE LARGER PORTIONS OF VEGETABLES AND LOW GLYCEMIC FRUITS.

YOU MAY HAVE ONE OR TWO AWARENESS MEALS A WEEK WHERE YOU CAN ENJOY A HAMBURGER, SOME PIZZA, OR ANOTHER FAVORITE FOOD. AN AWARENESS MEAL OCCURS WHEN YOU EAT WITH ATTENTION AND INTENTION. TAKE TIME BEFORE EATING THIS MEAL TO NOTICE IN-DEPTH THE COLORS, SHAPES, AROMAS, ETC. OF THE FOODS. WHILE EATING, CHEW DELIBERATELY AND NOTICE THE TEXTURES AND FLAVORS. RELISH EVERY BITE. IN ORDER TO MAINTAIN YOUR WEIGHT LOSS ACHIEVEMENT, HOWEVER, YOU MUST RETURN TO YOUR HEALTHY CLEAN LIFESTYLE TO KEEP HORMONAL BALANCE AND METABOLISM IN ORDER. DURING WEEK ONE, ONLY HAVE ONE AWARENESS MEAL, WEEK TWO HAVE TWO AWARENESS MEALS, WEEK THREE GO BACK TO ONE AWARENESS MEAL, AND WEEK FOUR HAVE TWO AWARENESS MEALS. THE POINT OF AN AWARENESS MEAL IS TO GIVE YOURSELF PERMISSION TO INDULGE IN SOME OF YOUR FAVORITE FOODS WITHOUT GUILT ONCE IN A WHILE. YOU DO NOT WANT TO BECOME ADDICTED TO PROCESSED FOODS SO THIS IS WHY AWARENESS MEALS SHOULD BE LIMITED. DURING PHASE1 AND 2, YOU BROKE YOUR ADDICTION TO PROCESSED FOODS SO DO NOT GO OVERBOARD ON YOUR AWARENESS MEALS.

YOU CAN ALSO CHOOSE THE BEST PROCESSED OPTIONS AS SHOWN ON THE SHOPPING TOUR.

PHASE 3 TIPS AND OVERVIEW

With PHASE 3, you can add foods back until you find yourself gaining weight or body fat percentage. This is where you jump back into PHASE 1 or 2 in order to reclaim your health. Remember health is a decision you make every day and every minute. You make decisions all the time. Always set goals for yourself and push yourself to improve. Encourage others to join you on the journey!

Finally here is a final review and some effective tips to becoming a master of healthy eating:

1. Know the 3 important blood sugar stabilization principles:
   - Eat a balanced meal every 3-4 hours.
   - Maintain balanced nutrient ratios at every meal (protein, fat, and carbohydrates).
   - Consume the correct amount of calories at each meal (based on metabolic rate testing).

2. Believe in the importance of QUALITY food:
   - Less ingredients on the label means less processing and slower digesting (less sugar spikes).
   - Eat food in a state closest to its NATURAL state (less cooked and refined).
   - Go for higher FIBER foods (more fiber slows digestion and less sugar spikes).
     - o Goal is around 45-50 grams a day.
     - o Take 15 grams in a supplement form twice a day with the rest from foods.

3. Less SODIUM means higher QUALITY:
   - Sodium makes you retain water leading to bloating and weight gain.
   - A bloated digestive system will not work properly leading to more weight gain.
   - Limit to less than 2,000 mg a day.

4. Follow mealtime guidelines:
   - 6:30 am   Meal 1: Breakfast - eat within 30-60 minutes of waking. If you are not hungry eat a half meal.
     The sooner you eat, the sooner the metabolism starts to work for you.
   - 9:30 am   Meal 2: Mid-morning meal
   - 12:30 pm   Meal 3: Lunch
   - 3:30 pm   Meal 4: Mid-afternoon meal
   - 6:30 pm   Meal 5: Dinner
   - 9:30 pm   Meal 6: Bedtime *Eat within one hour of going to bed to keep your metabolism firing through the night. If you are not hungry, eat a meal with only protein and fat.*

5. Avoid refined carbohydrates:
   - Pastas, breads, cereals, etc. are very broken down simple carbohydrates. Because they are quickly digested, they also cause a rapid blood sugar spike followed by a chaser of insulin trying to decrease the spike. As we know, with an insulin spike comes storage of fat and weight gain.

6. Focus on complete PROTEIN sources with meals:
   - Complete proteins have ALL the essential amino acids in them. Eating a complete protein first in your meal is the first step in blood sugar stability and thereafter weight loss.
   - Peanuts, peanut butter, nuts, and other nut butters are NOT a complete protein and not counted as protein.

PHASE 1 TIPS AND OVERVIEW

It can go towards your fat needs only.

7. If you get constipated with your higher complete protein intake, take more fiber and water:

    • You can do up to an additional 15 gram fiber supplement twice a day along with your other fiber. Too much fiber too quickly can also make you constipated. Start fiber slowly and work up to the recommended amount and always drink with plenty of water.

    • Take digestive enzymes and probiotics.

8. Optimize Meal Order:

    • Eat your protein first. It leads to a slower digestion rate of the entire meal.

    • Eat your fat second. Fat slows the acid release in stomach and slows digestion.

    • Eat your carbs last. This will allow the other nutrients to start digestion first which will release all the nutrients into the blood together and prevent blood-sugar spikes.

9. Design a MOBILE FOOD KIT:

    • Be careful not to miss a meal because it leads to sugar crashing and craving as well as slows metabolism. Have ON-THE-GO meals ready. They take little time to prepare leaving NO EXCUSES. A few good ideas include:

    o Apple and nuts
    o Protein bars
    o Protein drink
    o Greek yogurt
    o Cottage cheese with nuts and fruit
    o Low sodium deli meat with fruit
    o Edamame
    o Hard-boiled egg with fruit

10. Know what you can drink:

    • Caffeine

    o It will give you an energy burst followed by an energy crash. It also increases the Glycemic Index of all foods eaten which will lead to a higher insulin spike and fat storage in the end.

    o If putting caffeine back into meal planning after PHASE 1 or 2:

    o Limit to a.m. hours, take with food, avoid any high calorie (greater than 100 kcals) drinks, and factor calories into your meal planning.

    • Soda

    o No regular soda -They are all empty, fat forming, high glycemic index calories.

    o Diet soda (preferably decaf) - Take on occasion as to not make your mind and body crave more sweet flavors.

    • Alcohol

    o If taken in excess, it will slow the metabolism. Alcohol has a lot of calories without any nutrient value. Especially avoid at bedtime as it will cause an imbalance of your healthy sleep cycle. Limit to maximum

PHASE 1 TIPS AND OVERVIEW

of 2 or 3 drinks a week.

Realize that if you are not getting the body changes your desire, this MUST GO!

11. Use protein bars, powder, and/or drinks if needed:
   - They are second choice to real QUALITY protein foods.
   - They are good for on the go and convenience reasons.
   - Pick ones that have quality protein and a balance of the other nutrients.
   - Use a powder that is mostly protein without sugar and fat added.
   - Use a replacement a MAXIMUM of 2 meals a day. Try to get the rest from REAL food sources.

12. Enjoy a weekly OFF PLAN (awareness) meal:
   - This keeps you sane with something to look forward to during your week. It is important to find a "healthy" balance with this meal.
   - Eat consistently throughout the day on your awareness meal day; don't "store" up calories.
   - Make sure it is an experience and worth it. Go slowly and enjoy it fully to get the craving out of your system.
   - Jump back in to the West Clinic plan right after, and eat again within four hours to decrease the fat storage from the awareness meal. Leave out the carbs on this half meal.
   - Stay guilt free after your awareness meal. You deserved it and you are still on track!

   Again, this meal is not required for success. If you have the self-control and determination to stay "clean" the entire week that is great and you may achieve your results faster.

Here is a sample meal plan for PHASE 3. Feel free to use any of the recipes throughout this entire cookbook.

WEST CLINIC 4 LIFE PHASE 3:
1 MONTH OF EASY EATING WEEK 1

Sunday	Monday	Tuesday	Wednesday	Thursday	Friday	Saturday
Meal 1 Banana/ Peanut Butter	Meal 1 Kashi Go Lean/ Almond Milk/ Whey Protein	Meal 1 Smoothie: Strawberry/ Banana/ Va- nilla Whey Protein/ Almond Milk	Meal 1 Hard Boiled Egg/ Rice Cake/ Sun butter/ Sweet Peppers	Meal 1 Greek Yogurt/ Vanilla Whey/ Strawberries / Flax Seed	Meal 1 Grapefruit ½ c Cottage Cheese/ 5 Al- monds	Meal 1 1 Slice Whole Wheat Bread/ 1 Tbsp. Peanut Butter/ Orange
Meal 2 Celery Apple/ Whey Protein/ Rice Milk	Meal 2 10 Almonds/ Apple/ ½ Scoop Casein Protein	Meal 2 Apple/ Nat- ural Peanut Butter	Meal 2 ½ Apple/ ½ c Greek Yogurt/ 1 Tbsp. Walnuts	Meal 2 Cottage Cheese/ Fruit	Meal 2 2 Rice Cakes/ 1 Tbsp. Almond Butter	Meal 2 Hummus/ Veggies
Meal 3 Wrap/ Assorted Veggies/ Turkey	Meal 3 Bird's Eye Brown Rice & Veggies/ Tuna	Meal 3 Greek Yogurt/ Whey/ Vanilla Extract/ Berries/Bear Naked Low Sugar Gra- nola	Meal 3 Nut Thins/ Tuna or Chicken/ Veggies	Meal 3 Wrap/ Laughing Cow Cheese/ Chicken/ Buffalo Sauce/ Veggies	Meal 3 Brown Rice/ Beans/ Chicken/ Salsa	Meal 3 Cheat Meal
Meal 4 Triscuits/ Hummus/ Carrots	Meal 4 1 Tbsp. Avocado/ 3 Slices Turkey	Meal 4 Cooked Shrimp/ Light Co- conut Milk/ Steamed Veggies	Meal 4 Turkey/ String Cheese/ Veggies	Meal 4 Triscuits/ Hummus	Meal 4 Sweet Potato/ Olive Oil/ Cinnamon	Meal 4 Avocado/ Veggies/ Turkey
Meal 5 No Salt Canned Chicken/ Veggies/ Lettuce/Just Add Lettuce	Meal 5 Chicken/ Celery/ Greek Yo- gurt/ Ranch Flavor/ Lettuce	Meal 5 Rotisserie Chicken/ Mann's Mixed Veggies	Meal 5 Antioxidant Blend Steam- er Veggies/ Laughing Cow Cheese	Meal 5 Turkey/ Lettuce/ Sunflower Seeds/ Green Peppers	Meal 5 Tuna/ Celery/ Sweet Peppers/ Red Onion/ Cherry Toma- toes / Olive Oil	Meal 5 Lettuce/ Chicken/ Feta Cheese/ Olives/ Tomatoes / Just Add Lettuce Dressing
Meal 6 Casein Pro- tein/ Frozen Blueberries			Meal 6 Cottage Cheese			

WEST CLINIC 4 LIFE PHASE 3:
1 MONTH OF EASY EATING WEEK 2

Sunday	Monday	Tuesday	Wednesday	Thursday	Friday	Saturday
Meal 1 3 Egg whites/ Morning Star Sausage Patty/ Wrap/ Avocado	Meal 1 Shredded Wheat/ Milk/ Vanilla Whey Protein/ Banana	Meal 1 Greek Yogurt/ Walnuts/ Whey/ Blueberries / Low Sugar Bear Naked Granola	Meal 1 3 Egg Whites & 1 Full Egg/ Spinach/ Berries	Meal 1 2 Hard Boiled Egg Whites/ Sandwich Round/ Peanut Butter	Meal 1 Smoothie: Blueberries/ Raspberries/ Vanilla Whey Protein/ Milk	Meal 1 Quick Oats/Sun Butter/ Vanilla Whey Protein
Meal 2 2 Tbsp. Hummus/ Veggies/ Orange	Meal 2 Yogurt with Strawberries / Triscuits	Meal 2 Apple/ Peanut Butter	Meal 2 Triscuits/ Cottage Cheese	Meal 2 Almonds/ Fruit	Meal 2 String Cheese/ Nuts/ Apple	Meal 2 Cheat Meal
Meal 3 Wrap/ Hummus/ Turkey/ Olives/	Meal 3 Shrimp/ Greek Yogurt/ Chives/ Celery/ Wrap	Meal 3 Kashi Frozen Meal	Meal 3 Wrap/ Chicken/ Cabbage/ Pineapple/	Meal 3 Nut Thins/ Chicken or Tuna/ Onion/ Peppers/ Celery	Meal 3 Greek Yogurt/ Pineapple/ Whey	Meal 3 ½ Sandwich/ Turkey/ Lettuce/ Hummus/ Cucumbers/ Strawberries
Meal 4 Almond Breeze/ 1c Kashi Cereal/Flax	Meal 4 Protein Shake with Milk and Whey Protein	Meal 4 Hummus/ Triscuits	Meal 4 Protein Shake	Meal 4 Pure Protein Bar	Meal 4 Assorted Nuts/Granola/Just Fruit Dried Fruit	Meal 4 Cucumber/ Greek Yogurt Dill Dip
Meal 5 Assorted Nuts/Granola/Just Fruit Dried Fruit	Meal 5 Lettuce Wraps/ Boca Crumbles/ Peppers/ Onions/ Greek Yogurt	Meal 5 3 Hardboiled Egg Whites/ 1 Full Egg/ Raspberries	Meal 5 Coco Almonds	Meal 5 Lettuce/ Shrimp/ Egg/ Avocado/ Red Pepper	Meal 5 Cheat Meal	Meal 5 5 Egg Whites/ Veggies
Meal 6 Greek Yogurt Ranch Veggie Dip/ Mixed Veggies		Meal 6 Casein Protein/ Mixed Frozen Berries	Meal 6 Mann's Cauliflower mashed w/ Laughing Cow Cheese	Meal 6 Rotisserie Chicken/ Mann's Mixed Veggies	Meal 6 Cottage Cheese	Meal 6 Casein Protein/ Almonds

WEST CLINIC 4 LIFE PHASE 3:
1 MONTH OF EASY EATING WEEK 3

Sunday	Monday	Tuesday	Wednesday	Thursday	Friday	Saturday
Meal 1 Smoothie: Spinach/ Apples/ Kiwi/ Vanilla Whey Protein/ Milk	Meal 1 Quick Oats/Sun Butter/ Vanilla Whey Protein	Meal 1 Greek Yogurt/ Granola/ Blueberries/ Whey Protein	Meal 1 3 Egg whites/ Morning Star Sausage Patty/ Wrap/ Avocado	Meal 1 Rice Cake/ Sun butter/ Whey Protein/ Milk	Meal 1 Shredded Wheat/ Blueberries/ Flax Seed Powder	Meal 1 3 Egg Whites/1 Full Egg/ Almond Milk/ Banana
Meal 2 Greek Yogurt/ Almonds	Meal 2 String Cheese/ Turkey/ Nut Thins	Meal 2 2 Rice Cakes/ Almond Butter/ Veggies	Meal 2 Think Thin Protein Bar	Meal 2 String Cheese/ Apple	Meal 2 No Salt Canned Chicken/ Triscuits	Meal 2 Pure Protein Bar
Meal 3 Sandwich Round/ Turkey/ Mozzarella/ Lettuce	Meal 3 Tuna/ Brown Rice/ Birds Eye Mixed Veggies	Meal 3 Hummus/ Veggies/ Apple	Meal 3 Kashi Meal	Meal 3 Triscuits/ Hummus/ Veggies	Meal 3 Almonds/ Veggies/ Greek Yogurt w/ Ranch Seasoning	Meal 3 4 oz. Turkey/ Banana
Meal 4 Kashi Cereal/ Milk	Meal 4 Veggies/ Hummus/ Fruit	Meal 4 Assorted Nuts/Granola/Just Fruit Dried Fruit	Meal 4 Fruit/ Casein Protein	Meal 4 Detour Low Sugar Bar	Meal 4 Pure Protein Bar	Meal 4 Apple/ Peanut Butter
Meal 5 Sweet Potato/ Olive Oil/ Cinnamon	Meal 5 Mann's Cauliflower mashed w/ Laughing Cow Cheese	Meal 5 Rotisserie Chicken/ Mann's Veggies	Meal 5 1 lb Shrimp/ 1 Can Light Coconut Milk/ 1 tsp Curry/ Red Pepper Flakes/ Veggies	Meal 5 Cottage Cheese/ Sweet Peppers	Meal 5 Cheat Meal	Meal 5 No Salt Canned Chicken/ Triscuits
	Meal 6 Cottage Cheese	Meal 6 Casein Protein/ Almond Milk	Meal 6 Cottage Cheese/ Sunflower seeds	Meal 6 Greek Yogurt Ranch Dip/ Mixed Veggies	Meal 6 Casein Protein/ Walnuts	Meal 6 Cottage Cheese/ Almonds

WEST CLINIC 4 LIFE PHASE 3:
1 MONTH OF EASY EATING WEEK 4

Sunday	Monday	Tuesday	Wednesday	Thursday	Friday	Saturday
Meal 1 ½ Sandwich Round/ Peanut Butter/ Apple	Meal 1 3Egg Whites, 1 Full Egg/ Spinach Raspberries	Meal 1 Quick Oats/ Sun Butter/ Vanilla Whey Protein	Meal 1 Smoothie: Milk/ Greek Yogurt/ Vanilla Whey Protein/ Mixed Berries	Meal 1 Greek Yogurt/ Apple/ Walnut/ Nutmeg	Meal 1 Grape Nuts/ Hard Boiled Egg/ Blueberries	Meal 1 Shredded Wheat/ Milk/ Vanilla Whey Protein
Meal 2 Mann's Veggies/ Health Ranch	Meal 2 Pure Protein Bar	Meal 2 Think Thin Bar	Meal 2 Pure Protein Bar	Meal 2 Cinnamon Almonds	Meal 2 Greek Yogurt/ Pure Vanilla Extract/ Granola/ Vanilla Whey Protein/ Raspberries	Meal 2 Cinnamon Almonds/
Meal 3 Kashi Frozen Meal	Meal 3 Shrimp/ Birds Eye Rice Pilaf	Meal 3 Triscuts/ Laughing Cow Cheese	Meal 3 Kashi Meal	Meal 3 Mann's Veggies/ Brown Rice/ Chicken	Meal 3 Cheat Meal	Meal 3 Wrap/ Turkey/ Assorted Veggies/ Hummus
Meal 4 Tortilla, Blue Cheese Laughing Cow Light Cheese/ Pre Cooked Chicken, Buffalo Hot Sauce	Meal 4 Sea Salt Nut Thins/ Hummus	Meal 4 Mann's Veggies/ Hummus	Meal 4 3 Hardboiled Egg Whites/ 1 Full Egg/ Raspberries	Meal 4 Sun Butter/100% WW Bread/ Cinnamon	Meal 4 Pure Protein Bar	Meal 4 Sun Butter/100% WW Bread/ Cinnamon
Meal 5 Sweet Potato/ Cinnamon/ Olive Oil	Meal 5 Tuna/Wrap Tomato/ Lettuce/ Hummus	Meal 5 Almond Milk/Meal Replacement Shake	Meal 5 Apple/PB	Meal 5 Rotisserie Chicken/ Mann's Veggies	Meal 5 Pre-Cooked Chicken/ Salad/ Olive Oil Vinegar	Meal 5 Cheat Meal
Meal 6 Casein Protein/ Walnuts	Meal 6 Cottage Cheese	Meal 6 Greek Yogurt/ Dill/ Sweet Peppers	Meal 6 Casein Protein/ Coconut Milk	Meal 6 Mann's Cauliflower mashed w/ Laughing Cow Cheese	Meal 6 Cottage Cheese/ Almonds	Meal 6 Casein Protein/ Sunflower Seeds

GLUTEN FREE DIET GUIDE

A GLUTEN-FREE DIET IS RECOMMENDED FOR THOSE WITH AN ALLERGY OR INTOLERANCE TO WHEAT, RYE, OAT, BARLEY, KAMUT, TRITICALE, AND SPELT. ALTHOUGH MOST PEOPLE FOR WHOM A GLUTEN FREE DIET IS RECOMMENDED CAN TOLERATE OAT PRODUCTS, CROSS CONTAMINATION WITH WHEAT AND OTHER GRAINS CAN OCCUR IN BAKING. IF YOU USE OATMEAL OR STEEL CUT OATS, THE PACKAGE SHOULD SAY GLUTEN FREE. THOSE WITH CELIAC DISEASE ALSO FOLLOW A GLUTEN FREE DIET. BECAUSE YOU HAVE A GLUTEN INTOLERANCE OR ALLERGY DOES NOT MEAN YOU HAVE CELIAC DISEASE, HOWEVER THE DIET FOR BOTH IS SIMILAR.

IN ORDER TO CLEAR YOUR INFLAMMATION FROM YOUR GI TRACT, WE RECOMMEND YOU FOLLOW A GLUTEN FREE DIET FOR AT LEAST 3 MONTHS. FOR THOSE INDIVIDUALS WITHOUT A SEVERE ALLERGY TO GLUTEN, IT MAY BE POSSIBLE TO EAT SMALL AMOUNTS OF GLUTEN CONTAINING FOODS 1-2 TIMES A WEEK AFTER THE FIRST 3 MONTHS.

GLUTEN-FREE DIET FACTS

Foods that are acceptable on a gluten free diet:

Tolerable Grains	Corn	Wild Rice Rice	Fresh Fruits Fresh Vegetables	Lupine
Milk	Montina	Yams	Tapioca Millet	Arrowroot
Taro	Potatoes	Eggs	Sweet Potatoes	Nuts
Quinoa	Teff	Amaranth	Sorghum	

Gluten is frequently used as a stabilizing agent or a thickener in products like ice-cream and ketchups. Gluten can be found in over-the-counter or prescription medications, vitamins, and cosmetics such as lipstick, lip balms and lip gloss.

Avoid all ordinary breads, pastas, gravies, custards, soups, sauces, and many convenience foods.

Most grocery stores will have a section devoted to gluten free foods and some restaurants will have gluten free options.

Read food labels and avoid these foods:
Vegetable proteins and starch
Modified food starch
Malt flavoring
Glucose syrup
L-G

Some foods suggested by some of our patients:
- Bread - Udi is a multi-grain bread that is frozen
(Keep it in the freezer and take out one at a time to keep it moist)
- Bob's Red Mill (freeze the bread immediately after baking)
- Pamela's pancake mix
lutamine (as a supplement)   - Crunch Master

Crackers (Whole gluten free grains) Suggested Resources:
- Celiac Disease: A guide to living with Gluten Intolerance by Sylvia Bower
- Gluten Free grocery shopping guide by Matison and Matison (It is updated yearly).
- The Gluten Free Bible by Jax Peters Lowell.

Suggested Web sites:
http://www.mayoclinic.com/health/gluten-free-diet/MY01140
http://www.csaceliacs.org/gluten_grains.php

GLUTEN-FREE DIET FACTS

Gluten is another word for the proteins found in wheat, rye, and barley. Individuals with celiac disease must follow a gluten-free diet.

These gluten-free diet basics are important to know and follow.

<u>Wheat, rye, or barley</u>
Avoid wheat, rye, and barley. They all contain gluten.

<u>Oats</u>
Oats often are cross-contaminated with gluten-containing grains. Pure, uncontaminated oats, tested and labeled as gluten free, are now available and are considered safe to consume in moderation.

<u>Wheat and wheat-containing grains</u>
Other names for wheat or wheat-containing grains that contain gluten are:
• Spelt • Kamut® • Einkorn • Emmer • Triticale • Durum • Farina • Enriched flour • Wheat starch • Wheat germ
• Self-rising flour • Graham flour • Bulgur • Semolina • Cake flour • Pastry flour • Matzo

Wheat free does not mean gluten free. Wheat-free foods may still contain rye or barley.

<u>Malt</u>
Malt and malt flavorings are made from barley. They are not gluten free.

<u>Grains and flours that are safe</u>
The following grains and flours are safe for individuals on a gluten-free diet:
• Rice • Corn • Quinoa • Amaranth • Arrowroot • Buckwheat • Montina™ • Flax • Potato • Sago • Soy
• Sorghum • Tapioca • Teff • Cornstarch • Any flour made from nuts, beans, tubers, or legumes

<u>Cross contamination</u>
Follow this advice to prevent gluten-free foods from coming in contact with foods containing gluten:
• Store gluten-free foods separately from foods containing gluten.
• Designate certain appliances, such as a toaster, for use with gluten-free products only.
• Use clean tools for cooking, cutting, mixing, and serving gluten-free foods.
• Have separate containers of butter, peanut butter, and condiments, or institute a no-double- dipping rule.
• Do not purchase flour or cereal from open bins.

GLUTEN-FREE DIET FACTS

Foods to choose

Stick to plain, simple foods, which are mostly found in the outer aisle of the grocery store, including:

- All plain meats, poultry, fish, or eggs
- Legumes and nuts in all forms
- Corn and rice in all forms
- Dairy products, including milk, butter, margarine, real cheese, and plain yogurt
- All plain fruits or vegetables (fresh, frozen, or canned)
- Vegetable oils, including canola
- All vinegar, except malt vinegar
- Any food that says it is gluten free

References and recommended readings

Mahan LK, Escott-Stump S. Krause's Food and Nutrition Therapy. 12th ed. St. Louis, MO: Saunders/Elsevier; 2008.

National Digestive Diseases Information Clearinghouse (NDDIC). Celiac disease. Available at: http://digestive.niddk.nih.gov/ddiseases/pubs/celiac/. Accessed January 10, 2011.

Review Date 3/11 G-1536

Sunday	Monday	Tuesday	Wednesday	Thursday	Friday	Saturday
Meal 1 Banana and peanut butter or Sunbutter	Meal 1 ¼ c Bob's Red Mill GF Oats 1 Tbsp. ground flaxseed 1 Tbsp. craisins 1 tsp walnuts ½ scoop casein protein Cinnamon	Meal 1 Udi's Whole grain GF bread 2 egg whites Hummus	Meal 1 ½ c GF Oats ½ c cottage cheese 3 egg whites ½ c berries	Meal 1 3 egg whites Vegetable Fruit	Meal 1 1 Grapefruit ½ c Cottage Cheese 5 Almonds	Meal 1 1 GF Udi's whole grain bread 1 Tbsp. peanut butter or Sunbutter Orange
Meal 2 Whey protein (West Clinic's Dymatize Iso-100) Apple	Meal 2 10 Almonds Apple ½ scoop casein protein	Meal 2 Apple Natural Peanut Butter or Sunbutter	Meal 2 ½ apple ½ c Greek yogurt with walnuts	Meal 2 Cottage Cheese Fruit	Meal 2 2 Rice cakes 1 Tbsp. almond butter	Meal 2 Hummus and vegetable
Meal 3 GF Erewhon Brown rice cereal, rice milk or GF soymilk ½ c berries 2 Egg whites	Meal 3 2 C. Spinach 3 Oz. Tuna (Starkist is GF) Onion Green pepper Red pepper 1 Tbsp. balsamic vinegar 1 tsp. olive oil	Meal 3 Fage Greek Yogurt Ground Flax	Meal 3 ½ c Uncle Ben's brown rice 1 c veggies 1 chicken breast	Meal 3 Salad with chicken	Meal 3 1 GF (Food for Life) Brown rice tortilla wrap 3 oz. chicken breast 1c spinach 1/4c fat free cheddar cheese Mustard	Meal 3 Salad Tuna Cottage Cheese Fruit
Meal 4 GF Marys Gone Crackers GF Hummus Carrots	Meal 4 1 Tbsp. avocado 3 slices turkey(Hormel Natural is GF)	Meal 4 Spinach Arugula Broccoli Carrots Tuna Olive oil	Meal 4 Protein shake	Meal 4 Mary's Gone Crackers with Hummus	Meal 4 1Tbsp. avocado 3 slices turkey (Hormel Natural or Boars Head brands are GF)	Meal 4 Avocado Vegetable Turkey (Hormel)
Meal 5 Fage Greek yogurt Casein Protein (West Clinic's Dymatize Elite Casein) with cottage cheese	Meal 5 3 oz. sirloin Lots of carrots, peppers 1 Tbsp. hummus	Meal 5 Banana Whey protein with rice/soy milk	Meal 5 Salad with olive oil and vinegar Salmon fillet	Meal 5 Ground Turkey Vegetable ½ c sweet potatoes	Meal 5 3 oz. sirloin Carrots, peppers 1 Tbsp. hummus	Meal 5 Cheat Meal
	Meal 6 Cottage Cheese	Meal 6 Cottage cheese Almonds Turkey	Meal 6 Casein Protein/ Coconut Milk	Meal 6 Casein Protein Shake	Meal 6 Cottage Cheese Casein Protein	Meal 6 Casein Protein/ Sunflower Seeds

Sunday	Monday	Tuesday	Wednesday	Thursday	Friday	Saturday
Meal 1 Bobs Red Mill Steel cut oats Blueberries Protein Powder	Meal 1 GF Cereal ½ c soymilk Fruit	Meal 1 ½ Bobs Red Mill steel cut oats ½ sc choc. casein protein 1 tsp. peanut butter 1 tsp. flaxseed	Meal 1 Egg white Vegetables	Meal 1 3 egg whites Vegetable Fruit	Meal 1 ½ c GF oatmeal ½ c berries 1 scoop protein Walnuts	Meal 1 Egg White Omelet Udi's GF Bread Toasted
Meal 2 Apple with Natural peanut butter or Sunbutter	Meal 2 Mary's Gone Crackers Cottage Cheese	Meal 2 1 Tbsp. Hummus Vegetable	Meal 2 Yogurt with Blueberries/ Strawberries	Meal 2 Cottage Cheese Fruit	Meal 2 Almonds Fruit	Meal 2 Carrots Fage Greek Yogurt Garlic/Dill Seasoning
Meal 3 Spinach Salad with peppers, cucumbers, tomatoes, carrots	Meal 3 Sweet potato Tuna Salad	Meal 3 3 oz. beef sirloin Stir Fry: 2 c broccoli Red & green peppers 1/4c onion 1 Tbsp. GF Braggs amino acid 1c brown rice Red pepper flakes	Meal 3 Turkey Sandwich on GF Udi's Whole grain bread with Tomato Celery sticks with Natural Peanut Butter	Meal 3 Salad with chicken	Meal 3 GF Brown Rice Tortilla Salsa Chicken Vegetables	Meal 3 Brown Rice Tortilla Ham Mixed Vegetables Spinach Honey Mustard
Meal 4 Brown Rice Tortilla Lean beef (94/6) or Grass fed beef. Roasted Vegetables	Meal 4 Protein Shake	Meal 4 ½ c almond milk 1 c Brown Rice cereal	Meal 4 Cottage Cheese	Meal 4 Marys Gone Crackers with Hummus	Meal 4 Cucumber Fage Greek Yogurt Dip	Meal 4 Cottage Cheese Sweet Peppers
Meal 5 Casein Protein Shake	Meal 5 Chicken Breast Salad	Meal 5 Salad: 2 c romaine 2 oz. tuna 1.2 c cottage cheese Peppers onions	Meal 5 Chicken Breast Steamed vegetables Brown rice	Meal 5 Ground Turkey Vegetable ½ c sweet potatoes	Meal 5 Salmon Steamed Vegetables	Meal 5 Ground Turkey Lettuce Wrap
		Meal 6 Cottage cheese Almonds Turkey	Meal 6 Protein shake with skim milk, Whey protein and Vitamin C powder	Meal 6 Casein Protein Shake		Meal 6 Casein Protein/ Sunflower Seeds